Dyslexia

Dyslexia

A multidisciplinary approach

Edited by

Patience Thomson
MA, MEd
Principal of Fairley House

and

Peter Gilchrist
BA(TCD), MA(Child Psych), AFBPsS, C. Pyschol.
Consultant Educational Psychologist

Consultant Editors
Margaret Edwards
Jean Cooper
and
Robert Ringel

Stanley Thornes (Publishers) Ltd

First edition published in 1997 by Chapman & Hall

Reprinted in 2000 by:
Stanley Thornes (Publishers) Ltd
Ellenborough House
Wellington Street
Cheltenham
Glos.
GL50 1YW
United Kingdom

00 01 02 03 04 / 10 9 8 7 6 5 4 3 2 1

A catalogue record for this book is available from the British Library.
ISBN 0 7487 5793 7

Typeset by Mews Photosetting, Beckenham, Kent
Printed and bound in Great Britain by Athenæum Press Ltd, Gateshead, Tyne & Wear

Contents

Contributors

Angela Dominy
BEd, DipRSA(SpLD)
Class teacher

Peter Gilchrist
BA(TCD), MA(Child Psych), AFBPsS, C. Psychol.
Educational Psychologist

Ingrid Linge
BSc, SROT
Occupational Therapist

Vivienne McKennell
MA, CQSW
School Counsellor

Nicholas Rees
MA, PGCE, DipRSA(SPld)
Class teacher

Jeanne Reilly
DipCST, CertEdAd, MCSLT
Speech and Language Therapist

Patience Thomson
MA, MEd,
Headteacher

Sam Tucker
MBBCH, FRCP, FRCPE, DCH
Consultant Paediatrician

Ann Wilson
MBE, DBO(T)
Orthoptist

Foreword by Sir Roger Bannister

This book is written by the Headteacher and the Educational Psychologist of Fairley House, a school for dyslexic children, and their staff and includes contributory chapters from staff and colleagues associated with the school. They have as much expertise as any group in the country. It is enjoyable to read because of the authors' dedication and a touch of humour shines through its pages, enlivened by vivid case reports. The basic theme of the book is that the multidisciplinary approach described here is necessary to rescue dyslexic children from the burden of their frustration.

Dyslexia is indeed a puzzling phenomenon. How astonishing it is that when the word '19' is spoken to some dyslexics it may be written as 91, 61 or even 16. Learning language is of course the secret of the human race's ascent of the evolutionary ladder but this book shows us that it is still a wonder that any of us manage to read or write at all. The reason we do learn is that most children are enormously adaptable, even overcoming the difficulties of poor schools and broken homes. I like the little boy whose only seeming interest was a shyly declared wish to play the guitar. It was this link that led him back to living again. Nothing, as they say, succeeds like success, any success, and when it happens it is as if a light goes on in their young lives.

My own personal interest in dyslexia was triggered some 30 years ago, with colleagues at the National Hospital for Neurology and Neurosurgery in London, by the problems of the crossed-laterality of the dyslexic. This book describes the separation of this discrete group of orthoptic contributory factors and underlines the basic theme of the book – a multidisciplinary approach. It is not easy for the Health Service eye clinic or optician to gain the experience that this book will teach them and so correct a visual problem quickly and let more subtle management of the language problem start.

In many areas of dyslexia, practice and management have now outstripped neurological theory, though this in time may catch up.

Perhaps in the future the positron emission scanners will show how the right hemisphere precedes the left in language learning but for the present Patience Thomson and her team, and others like them, offer the best hope in this confusing field. Even they frankly admit to disappointment and occasional failure. But it is clear that if the team's experience is applied in assessing children over the course of a day before accepting them, then their own techniques can help most of the children whom they select. In some instances, they can be transformed from hopelessly confused children, bullied and losing friends at school, rejected by ordinary teachers and sometimes by parents, difficult, unruly, untidy, disobedient, disorganized and hopeless. I can think of nothing more satisfying than the pleasure of rescuing such children who have lost all self-esteem. If one can produce a child who can cope and sometimes release frustrated talents it is an astonishing transformation.

In this book the children and their parents have the last word. Mark said, 'It wasn't that I didn't have ideas or lack knowledge. Homework for others was 90% of the time spent on thought and 10% on writing. I spent 90% of my time thinking how to write it down and 10% writing it down wrongly'. This book deals with the dyslexic problem in the context of the family as well as the school. Mothers loom larger than fathers in the picture but as one paediatric physican said, 'A parent is a terrible thing to waste'. Parents in their way, and in particular mothers, reorganize their lives around the problems of their dyslexic children. Winnicott praised the concept of the 'good enough' mother and, one might add, father too. The mothers speak from the heart with blunt candour. 'I could cheerfully strangle every person who, learning of Peter's dyslexia, said "Look how well Susan Hampshire has done". Another mother summed it all up: 'Until I learnt to accept my child as a whole with his difficulties being part and parcel of his personality, I was in essence part of the problem'. Another said, 'It was only when Jack made the deliberate and absolute decision to deprive himself of his nightly story that I realized that he had considered obliterating the idea that words could bring pleasure for him; they brought pressure and punishment. But he knew he needed them and therein also lay pain'.

The cruel jibe that dyslexia was an excuse to shield lazy or inadequate children should now never be heard agian. It is a tragedy that there are still many children whose problems are not being seriously addressed. It is my fervent hope that the book will be a beacon not only to those already interested in the field but also to education authorities all over the country. State schools should have state funding for specialized teaching. In my view no school of any standing should be without this volume, so that many children who are still in deep trouble can be rescued.

I would predict that this book will become a classic for similar teams of teachers of dyslexics and indeed for all teachers of children and all parents of dyslexics. I wish it the success it richly deserves.

Roger Bannister

Acknowledgements

We would like to thank the following for material which has been included in the various chapters of this book: Maggie Percival, Sally Sinclair, Rosena Mentior, Caroline Lillywhite, Wendy Mountford, Jenny Dromgoole, Carrie Beaumont, Peter Cross, Mel Lever and Hannah Fussner and other members of staff for helpful advice, painstaking proofreading and general encouragement, especially Juliet Lambert.

We would also like to thank the children and parents for their substantial contributions to Chapter 1 of the book and for ideas and insights throughout.

Finally we would like to make grateful mention of the untiring patience of Anne Fitzgerald and Louise Austin who typed the major part of the manuscript.

This book is dedicated to staff, pupils and parents, past and present, and to Daphne Hamilton-Fairley, without whose inspiration and determination there would have been no Fairley House School.

To preserve confidentiality the parents and children who contributed to Chapter 1 have been given pseudonyms. For the same reason the names in the case studies presented in the book have been changed.

The masculine pronoun ('he', 'him') is used in the text to refer to any child. This is merely to aid readability and should not be taken to imply that only male children are being discussed.

1   *Dyslexia – whose problem?*

Patience Thomson

Introduction

This book was commissioned to illustrate how a multidisciplinary team, working in one particular location, interacts in the diagnosis and management of a particular problem – dyslexia or specific learning difficulties. Its content may be of considerable interest to teachers and members of the lay public, including parents, who have an interest in the subject. Its primary purpose, however, is to convey to professionals in fields related to the management of specific learning difficulties the impact which can be made by the intervention of a well-integrated multidisciplinary team.

The professionals contributing chapters to this book had a clearly defined brief, which was to rationalize and describe their actual role, the significance of their input and the framework of cooperation with their colleagues to provide comprehensive support for the dyslexic child.

One obvious hazard in approaching a topic such as dyslexia in this way is that it may appear too insular. Could the working relationships and remedial programmes established in a specialist school like Fairley House be replicated elsewhere? A school established as a charitable foundation with about 100 dyslexic children of primary school age, staying on average no more than two or three years and with a pupil:staff ratio of 3:1, is scarcely a typical educational environment. The value of the book lies in the conviction that there are significant general conclusions which can be drawn from the experience of this particular institution.

What emerges strongly is the benefit of a holistic approach. When this is achieved, it is astonishing to discover how many factors affect progress, all of which must be considered if the child's problems are to be addressed in the most effective way possible. Not all these factors are strictly educational in nature. They are nonetheless important because they enable the child to develop the skills and attitudes which will be as crucial as an educational remedial programme in overcoming the difficulties created by dyslexia.

Without the attributes of self-control, strong motivation, enthusiasm, persistence and self-respect, progress will inevitably be slow. Can such attributes be acquired through teaching, therapy and example? Can interpersonal skills such as the ability to learn from others, to listen, to communicate and to work cooperatively be incorporated successfully in the overall plan? What effects do these factors have on the child's ability to learn? These are some of the important issues which are explored by experts from different disciplines in this book.

The dyslexic conundrum

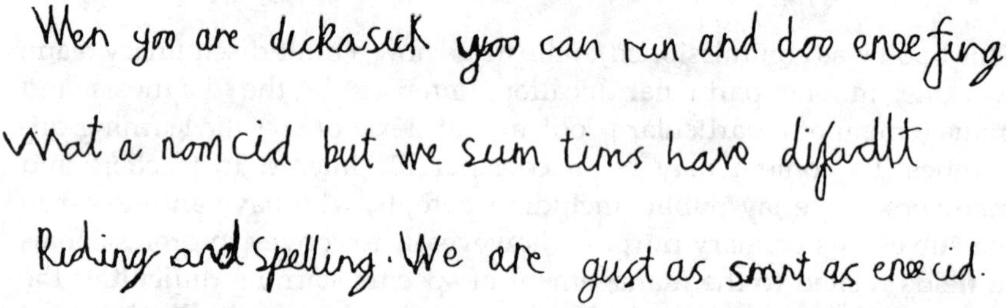

When yoo are dickasieck yoo can run and doo enoe fing Wat a nom cid but we sum tims have difadlt Riding and Spelling. We are gust as smrt as enoe cid.

Fig. 1.1 Definition of dyslexia by a 10-year-old boy.

Dyslexia is a puzzling phenomenon and a precise definition is elusive. The term 'specific learning difficulties', which is often used as an alternative, can be helpful because it implies problems in certain identifiable areas rather than global impairment. It also embraces the term 'dyspraxia', discussed at length in Ingrid Linge's chapter. Children of relatively low ability are described as having mild, moderate or severe learning difficulties. Dyslexic children do not fall into any of these categories. They have discrepant difficulties, strengths and often pronounced weaknesses, which alternatively astonish or dismay parents and teachers. Most of all they are confused themselves, receiving constant mixed messages. Their pattern of difficulties is complex and can vary quite markedly in different individuals.

Dyslexic children are vulnerable in certain crucial areas. These can include the auditory and visual processing of sounds and symbols, organization and sequencing, directionality and orientation and expressive and receptive language, especially where written work and information processing are concerned. Social behaviour can be affected. If we include within the term 'specific learning difficulties' problems with gross and fine motor control, then problems with coordination, balance and body image also enter the picture. Dyspraxic children will have problems with conceptualizing, planning and executing motor tasks and may appear clumsy or careless.

What problems does dyslexia create?

Difficulties in the areas described above create problems not only at school but at home. At school they prevent the easy acquisition of the basic literacy skills of reading, writing and spelling and extend into many other areas of the curriculum. Most teaching, in any subject, involves communication through language. A language deficit must therefore constitute a major handicap. The dyslexic child cannot do justice to his ability and is often underestimated or accused of being unmotivated or lazy. The ensuing effect on morale can lead to emotional or behavioural problems including aggressive tendencies, withdrawal or avoidance strategies. Such difficulties will almost always dent the child's self-respect and lead to frustration and lack of confidence. At home the child's apparently disappointing academic performance and negative attitude to school will leave parents concerned and anxious. Homework may become an embattled nightmare.

Dyslexic children are often not 'unacademic' but their difficulties in learning how to read effectively debar them from accessing many of the usual sources of information. As they grow older, this inability may be a cause of shame and invite the mockery of classroom peers. We live in a society where literacy skills are all too often equated with intelligence. It is small wonder that they show little enthusiasm for school if they are constantly exposing themselves to humiliation and ridicule.

Dyslexics are often accused of having poor concentration. Those who are not musical can empathize with the problems of the dyslexic by comparing the position of the child with language-processing difficulties with that of an unmusical member of the audience at a concert. If the music is unfamiliar, if the pattern and structure of the piece are unrecognized and the person in question hears noise rather than melody, the mind will switch off and occupy itself with plans, practicalities or fantasies. In the same way dyslexic children will switch off in school, since a poor auditory memory and weak sequencing skills cause them to lose the thread of the lesson. They fail to understand the written comments on the board or in the textbook and struggle to make continuing sense of what the teacher is saying. Finally they lose interest, cease to exert themselves and resort to diversionary tactics or retire into their own private world.

Unfortunately for these children, competent literacy and numeracy skills are almost essential for success in modern life. Qualifications are needed for most careers. Many dyslexics will be debarred from jobs in areas where they have the potential to succeed because they will be seriously disadvantaged in tests and examinations. If they are of average intelligence or above and are going to profit from secondary education or beyond, it is a matter of real urgency that they should learn to read, write and spell and master the basic concepts of maths before they leave their primary school. If this is to happen their problems must be addressed as early as possible. Because of the diversity and complexity of their difficulties, this can be best achieved through the intervention of a multidisciplinary team.

Towards a practical definition of dyslexia

It is important to establish what is meant by the term 'dyslexia' within the context of this book. This will be done implicitly throughout by practical examples, case studies and the comments of experienced professionals working in the field, rather than by attempting to formulate a theoretical definition or quoting widely from the research literature. Brief mention, however, needs to be made at this early stage of both historical perspective and current opinion to explain how the concept of 'dyslexia' has broadened to embrace a wider spectrum of specific learning difficulties, with important implications for diagnosis and management.

Dyslexia has attracted the attention of a number of different professional disciplines and was, in fact, originally identified by those working in the medical field, who described the clinical features of the syndrome. In 1895, James Hinshelwood, a British ophthalmologist, became interested in the case of acquired dyslexia, where a man had lost the ability to read. Hinshelwood subsequently established that there were individuals whose dyslexia (or 'word blindness' as he called it) was congenital in origin.

Samuel Orton, in the United States, was a doctor with a particular interest in psychiatry and neurology. He described some of the classic symptoms of the dyslexic child, such as reversal of letters, syllables and words, left–right confusion and mixed lateral dominance, and associated them with a functional brain disorder. He broadened the definition of dyslexia from a reading problem to a more comprehensive interpretation of the syndrome and included disorders in the areas of both speech and language and motor planning.

Samuel Orton became an immensely influential figure in introducing the concept of dyslexia to both the medical and the educational world. He was interested in both the identification of a 'specific language difficulty', or dyslexia, and its practical management.

The Orton Society, whose annual meetings constitute an important international forum in this field, adopted a useful working definition of dyslexia in 1994.

> Dyslexia is a neurologically based, often familial, disorder which interferes with the acquisition and processing of language. Varying in degrees of severity, it is manifested by difficulties in receptive and expressive language, including phonological processing, in reading, writing, spelling, handwriting, and sometimes arithmetic. Dyslexia is not the result of lack of motivation, sensory impairment, inadequate instructional or environmental opportunities, or other limiting conditions, but may occur together with these conditions. Although dyslexia is lifelong, individuals with dyslexia frequently respond successfully to timely and appropriate intervention.

The British Dyslexia Association also redefined 'dyslexia' in 1989 as:

> A specific difficulty in learning, constitutional in origin, in one or more of reading, spelling and written language, which may be accompanied by difficulty in number work. It is particularly related to mastering and using a written language (alphabetic, numerical and musical notation) although often affecting oral language to some degree.

It is interesting to note that this definition broadens the concept of a 'lexical' difficulty by including numerical symbols and musical notation. Many would say, however, that both these definitions are incomplete. In an article entitled 'Can there be a single definition of dyslexia?', Elaine Miles (1995) writes:

> Dyslexia is not the sort of concept that can be summed up in a single formula; for different purposes different facets of dyslexia need to be mentioned. As all these may be valid, 'description' may be a better term to use than 'definition'. There is confusion as to how the word is actually used in practice and this has affected research.

Given the difficulties of producing a clearcut definition, it is hardly surprising that statistics vary as to the incidence of dyslexia among the general population. Moreover, the symptoms fall into a continuum, with some individuals far less severely affected than others. Research into the whole area of specific learning difficulties has produced many new insights into the multifarious factors which create specific learning difficulties, but it has not always been conclusive. However, the challenges offered by research to any preconceived ideas and the changing perspectives it affords are essential ingredients in preventing any institution involved in the dyslexic field becoming inflexible, insular or self-satisfied.

There is still much to be learned about dyslexia from both the medical and the educational perspective.

Margaret Rawson, now in her nineties, looks back over 55 years of involvement in the field of dyslexia and writes:

> The question of a definition for the term 'Dyslexia' must be addressed. There are some concepts, like language itself, of which it can be said that everybody knows what it is, but no one has been able to present a wholly satisfactory definition of it. Experience has convinced me that dyslexia is such a concept. The best that one can do in such a case is to name what one is talking about and then describe it with an appropriate explanatory purpose or viewpoint. One such view might be the centre of interest to the describer, while another could be an attempt to cast the description into the verbal language comfortable to one's respondent, whether colleague or audience.
>
> (Rawson, 1995)

In practical terms the definition of the word 'dyslexia' varies according to the discipline and perceptions of the person using it and of their audience, whether these are educational psychologists, speech and language therapists, occupational therapists, teachers, parents, children, local authority representatives or members of the general public.

Elaine Miles' proposal that a 'description' can in many cases prove more helpful than a 'definition' has the advantage that it can be more broadly based. If a description rather than a definition is required, dyslexics can themselves comment perspicaciously on the nature and extent of their problems and can detail the practical consequences.

Mark (Adult)

It wasn't that I didn't have ideas or lack of knowledge, it was that I could not get my thoughts across on paper. It always seemed strange to me that people appeared to write without thinking, while I was fighting for each word, trying to piece it together in my mind, trying to imagine what it looked like and still getting it wrong. Most of the time I wasn't thinking about the subject or text but simply 'How do I form this word?' Of course this meant that homework, notetaking and exams took far longer than they should. For others, 90% of the time was spent on thought and 10% writing it down – I spent 90% of my time thinking how to write it down and 10% writing it down wrong. For instance in notetaking, I would always be at least a board behind, as I memorized each word and its spelling and copied it down, rather than memorizing each complete sentence and then writing it down knowing the spelling already. It also meant I thought only about the form of the words and not what they meant.

Again, in homework, I would endlessly search for the right way to phrase the answer and still have to spend as much time as everyone in thinking about the answer.

But the biggest battles were examinations which, at the end of my tests, were so covered in red ink one was unable to see the blue ink. Any mistakes I read as right, and even missing words I would read as there – so the number of times I read through the piece was immaterial.

In reading I am less full of memories as my difficulties started very early on. What I do remember is reading word by word and with each word I would try to spell out how it sounded and then, on managing a reasonable attempt, I would search my memory for something which sounded verbally similar. By the time I reached the end of the sentence I couldn't remember what the words had all meant and so staggered through the sentence again and again until I had learnt it off by heart. By that stage I was already losing interest.

After learning to write my numbers the correct way round, arithmetic proved the easiest of the 3Rs, but even that had its problems with small mistakes continually cropping up, especially under pressure. I can remember once posting an urgent letter to number 15 instead of 51. But it was a grasp of essential arithmetic which inspired me to read my first book and won me my first wager. Having never read a page before, my mother made me an offer. 'If you can read a page,' she said, 'I will give you a penny and double it each time you read another page'. Well, there were only two reasons I stopped at £40.96. The first was that it was enough to buy a bike, the second was that I had reached the end of the book.

Teaching is a question of clarity. I think all pupils dislike ideas which are thrown at them in a disorganized way. They like ideas to be presented so that they can interconnect them and relate them to the subject. I had great difficulty at first, and still do, in re-sorting and organizing facts so that I had formed a basis and understanding of the subject before I moved on in it.

I will now move onto the social problems I encountered and still do to some extent encounter. I think all children can tell if another child is different, even though they don't know what that difference is. Every child gets teased a little, but I could have written books on the number of nicknames I collected. Some of them were to do with work and it didn't help when teachers classed me as lazy and careless.

It often seemed a hopeless struggle as I never seemed to improve however hard I tried. My family can testify to the tantrums I used to fly into when I felt the whole world was against me, and the times I would pack my rucksack and leave home.

Many dyslexics would empathize with what Mark is saying. Others would distance themselves and would question the severity of his dyslexic problem in view of the reasonable level of academic achievement manifested in his clear account of his problems. They could well feel that their own struggle had been more intense and more disheartening and that their difficulties had been less satisfactorily resolved.

Individual feelings about dyslexia

CHILDREN

A dyslexic adult, particularly one who has learned the strategies to cope with many of his specific difficulties, can look back with some equanimity and humour at his past struggles. Children may be less objective, but can also describe with clarity and feeling how dyslexia has affected many aspects of their lives. In this opening chapter it seems appropriate to allow the children themselves and their parents to make some contribution towards an understanding of what dyslexia means to the individual child and to the family.

The first three samples of the children's comments are general in nature. The standard of literacy varies considerably, but the underlying themes are the same.

Sam (10)

A year earlier, Sam was a non-starter in both reading and writing. He had such weak communication skills that he found talking to adults a painful experience, to be avoided whenever possible.

I finer it hrd to rit
I finer it hrd to sdrt (start) wat to rit. I finer it hrd to fingck (think)
I finer it hrd to cachat (concentrate)
I finer it hrd to remebfings (remember things)

Sally (10)

Sally listed her difficulties with some coherence:

1. organizing myself for school & enthing els.
2. I find it hard to conontrat (concentrate) wen I am not in goiing (enjoying) the leson.
3. homework. Wen I am at hom it is harder than school.
4. I hat (hate) to rit.
5. I have difrent problems eche day.
6. allathow (although) you wod thinck your wont get teast but ...

Martin (11)

Martin chose to treat the subject autobiographically.

Duing my life so far I have had some prety big knokes. First I went to my nersry where I probly had my worst experaince becaues my teacher thought not only I was stupid but that I never tried. When in reality I was trying so hard. The kids made it worse, they would go off and wisper about me and sunddnly look at me with diserproving look as if I had no perpers in this world or I am a wast of human resorces. I moved onto a school which was my worst nightmare. I spent threee hours doing my home work and I was really pleased with it So the next day I went to school real conferdent and then when I handed my home work in and the teacher just took one look and then tore it up. I was so dismayed that I nearly broke down in tears.

  By the time I was seven I was a nevers wreak who had so much agretion that I could explode.

Several other children wrote with a mixture of pain and anger about lack of understanding from teachers and their peers in previous, mainstream schools.

Samantha (10)

I used to say to myself. You know this well why can't you do it? as it was I had lernt it but the answer was somewhere in a room I was unable to unlock. My comunication was bad. I could not get the right words across to the other person and sometimes they just walked away. It's like (in the brain) when your trying to find the right words to say. It's exactly like someone switching of a light or taking out a plug and there is one think I can't explain 'How annoying it is!!'.

Robert (11)

The boys were often more resentful than the girls.

I think that being dislexsik is hard to live with if you don't have the write help. When I was in one of the speling classes at my old school the teacher would go arerend the class and jusy suddenle pount at them and egspect them to spell out the word that she said. If I had gone to a nother school like that one they would have probly stuck a big fat sine one my report saying DUMB!

Other people's lack of understanding of the implications of dyslexia extends to all areas of a child's life. It results in inhibitions, frustrations and a general wariness of being 'shown up' or ridiculed in any group situations either at school or at home, within or outside the family.

Social problems and the inability to establish or maintain friendships, 'unfair' criticism and negative differential treatment are far more common themes than academic frustrations and difficulties.

Naomi (11)

Naomi was determined to be honest because she wanted to be sure that her message got through.

I have been and still am dyslesia and dyspraxia. I was called stupid and dum and I was so distressed I would eat for comfort. But the thing that really buged me was that my best friend had a enormasly hye I que people would say how could you be her best friend this hurt me so I nilly ran away. And on one ocation I loked myself in the bathroom. People would say I was fat but it wasnt my fault. I was seven when I new I was dyslexia. people would say there gose fatty she is so lazzy and fat she dosnt belong in ur world she poluts are planet.

Tessa (11)

It felt like everyone hated me children were agants me Teachers were agants me. I was told I couldent do eny thing. When I hatto (had to) copy of the bord I never finished and all the spellings were always rong, my marks were low and I got told of for it. They used to sit me in a corner so I wouldent disturb or copy people and I was never chosen to answer question.

James (11) and Ian (10)

Several children reported behaviour which they knew was out of line, but which they felt unable to control. James and Ian are classmates. James was quite conscious that he was irritating to teach, just as Ian knew that his behaviour was not acceptable.

James:

I dont no wot to rite. I fgit (forget) things the brol (whole) time and I find it hud to stut sunting (start something) and I sing in class my Teacher finds it very frustrating I can not constranting. I hast (have) to say sili coments.

Ian:

For some reasen I sometimes get out of hand. I fined consanthating (concentrating) very hard and I fined being sensebol (sensible) hard to.

Clare (10)

Clare was equally honest, but for a different reason.

I do my homewoke with my mum and if my homework is hard I shrem (scream) and chawet (shout) at her. If I am toled to be uwiut (quiet) at school I chawet (shout) at my teacher and I tale her to be wriut (quiet).

John and Andrew (both 12)

John and Andrew mention avoidance strategies. Feeling ill was one and covering up or lying about inadequacies was another. John had evolved his own technique:

In the end I resorted to feeling ill about four times a week.

Andrew covered up his problems:

I can remember ling (lying) about not beeing bad at a subject, saing I cand do somthinck wick I cad not do.

If children mentioned their academic difficulties at all, there was a general consensus that reading and spelling had presented problems; some focused on other specific areas including handwriting and maths.

Edward and John (both 12)

Two boys told jointly of their hatred of mental arithmetic. It was a measure of their vulnerability that their reaction to the prospect of failure was so violent.

Edward:

In maths we have a thing called mental arithmetic. We all hate it and are going to tell you are feelings on it. It gets you soo cross you code give up come pletly and be depest.

John:

In school we have to do mental arithmetic. When I do it for home work I get rely stress and even give up and smash all my Lego modls.

Memory problems and difficulties with information processing were mentioned not infrequently as significant sidelines in the text. 'I feget things in a scond or two.' 'I foget what the teacher say. And I don't udsty (understand) my teacher.'

In summary, there was much evidence that the children were sensitively aware of their problems and could identify them with precision and clarity. The comments also highlighted their sense of vulnerability and helplessness and revealed how the nature of their difficulties provoked anxiety over a wide range of daily activities.

PARENTS

The central theme in many of the letters from parents is the way in which family dynamics are affected by the problems of the dyslexic child. Parents expressed themselves as concerned, anxious, frustrated and sometimes guilt ridden. They are angry at the lack of suitable help available. Many parents speak of the negative implications for them in terms of both time and money. Often sensitivity, empathy and understanding are displayed, especially in families where there is a genetic history of dyslexia. There is an underlying sense of pride that their children have had the courage and determination to overcome their difficulties and their positive qualities and achievements are emphasized.

Several parents explain how they have had to readjust their sights and revise their expectations. Even at this early stage, they are anxious about the children's future job prospects in a highly competitive world. There is, however, a general sense of relief that the diagnosis and identification of specific learning difficulties at least make it possible to plan realistically and to understand what must be achieved before the child can hope to compete on more equal terms with his non-dyslexic peers.

These extracts from parents' letters are self-explanatory.

Peter's mother

The effect on the entire family of the youngest child being dyslexic has been quite dramatic and will obviously be a lifelong issue. Peter was not diagnosed as dyslexic until he was well into his eighth year. However, the frustration and awkwardness of not fitting in or being like other children has been with Peter from a very early age and this resulted in over-reaction to almost every situation and made him feel forlorn and something of a misfit.

In addition to the above, he was badly bullied in several schools and the fact that he moved schools so often clouded the issue of his real disabilities.

We are still at the stage of being immensely regretful that Peter has learning difficulties and this has strengthened our resolve, which is natural to every parent, to help him overcome these and make his own way in life. Naturally we will not expect too much or too little of him, as with all his brothers and sisters we understand that every child and eventually every person finds their own niche and level in life.

It has opened our eyes to the huge range of difficulties associated with dyslexia throughout our culture and people's perceptions of them. I could quite cheerfully strangle every person who, upon learning of Peter's dyslexia, says, 'Look how well Susan Hampshire has done'.

Thomas's mother

Thomas is very cross and anxious about being dyslexic. 'I wish I could live in someone else who wasn't dyslexic. I'd like to take my brain out and make the two sides the same. Do I have a brain or is that it just doesn't work?' He sees dyslexia as a barrier to achieving a good job (highly paid!). It's prevented him from taking his rightful place in the family. He is the eldest of four children and as such in his eyes he should be best at everything – older brothers are supposed to know more or be able to do things better than younger ones. His pride and self-esteem take a double knock, not only does he have to grapple with the problem (as he puts it) of not being as good as or as clever as his friends, he sees his younger brother overtaking him. Nevertheless Thomas can get very cross and aggressive with his younger bother if he lets him down.

Thomas's answer to all this:

1. Convincing us that he's not interested in any of the things that he's not good at. (This charade has gone on for so long he may

have managed to convince himself). He used to manifest his frustration physically by tearing the offending piece of work up.

2.   Holds back – unless he's entirely sure he's going to be successful he will not tackle or be seen to tackle a task. We are not allowed to see him putting effort into tasks which he finds difficult. He always tries to make it appear that homework is easy and doesn't require much effort.

3.   Decided to become an expert in something he thinks is unrelated to things we value or know anything about or thinks dyslexia cannot prevent him from achieving.

How it affects the family:

Very easy to misunderstand behaviour caused by dyslexia and lash out. It's not so easy to treat it fairly and constructively and understand that fear, frustration, short-term memory problems and lack of motor control or spatial awareness are often the reasons – not naughtiness and spitefulness. It could be a potential minefield for dissension among adults – parents, uncles, aunts, brothers and sisters.

Ralph's mother

How Dyslexia has Affected our Son and the Family as a Whole

His poor self-esteem and frustration caused by his learning difficulties have been a cause for concern for his teachers as well as his parents. He has lost many of his original school friends because he could not relate to them in a socially acceptable way.

The initial struggle to have his difficulties identified and the constant battle to secure an appropriate education have proved extremely distressing to the whole family.

Naomi's mother

After losing a first pregnancy, Naomi was a precious first child. She was particularly demanding as a baby and like most new and inexperienced parents we doted on her.

My husband and I had two other sets of friends who also had daughters within weeks of Naomi's birth, but although she thrived physically, she never made the same progress as the other babies did. There was no competition, but Naomi seemed to come last in everything – last to roll, sit and walk. As parents we felt we were failing her and doing something wrong.

Naomi was finally diagnosed as being dyslexic at the age of six and to say it changed our lives is an understatement. For one thing my husband recognized himself from suffering from the same symptoms and was delighted to put his own lack of academic achievement down to dyslexia.

We could now explain that our slightly 'odd child' was different because her learning mechanism was defective, but Naomi looked very normal and everyone expected her to behave normally. Having an invisible handicap, I found myself protecting her to an absurd degree. In company I made jokes of her strange pieces of conversation to divert attention. I cringed at her inability to make eye contact, her unreasonable temper tantrums, her very poor interpersonal skills, never quite being 'tuned in', and her inability to learn the simplest of tasks, let alone literacy and numeracy skills.

Despite explaining Naomi's difficulties, her younger sister never really understood. Beyond sibling rivalry, she had been impatient with her, but could never understand why she needed so much help. Life for Naomi and her family has been an uphill struggle.

The greatest hurdle my husband and I had was adjusting our own expectation of our children. There is no doubt that many of us go into parenthood with very preconceived ideas of how we will bring up our families. It comes as a very rude awakening to discover that real life is just not like that.

Tamsin's father

We know our children are tall or skinny or clumsy perhaps, but dyslexia has few physical signs.The process by which most parents become aware of it is painful – not least for the dyslexic child.

We sent our second child to school full of hope for the future. This child, who talked early and who was bright and enthusiastic, did well enough at kindergarten and in the early years of 'proper school'. Slowly, almost imperceptibly, the progress reduced until we knew, but still doubted we even knew, that something was wrong. School was hell and homework was a nightmare. Worse than that, the happy child we had known had gone. Our daughter was sullen, sulky and difficult to communicate with. The outgoing, cheerful child had lost her spark. Friendliness had been replaced with diffidence. Restful sleep was interrupted by violent nightmares. Enthusiasm was hard to find and reluctance the order of the day. The change was not rapid, but its slowness made it no more comprehensible.

The visit we subsequently made to an educational psychologist was an enlightenment. We were surprised – 'She has difficulty in copying from the blackboard, doesn't she?' said the psychologist. She does, but how did he know? He knew because the systematic testing methods he used were well researched. He was able to rationalize the difficulties she (and we) had encountered. We had come to understand and identify specific learning difficulties.

For two years we have benefited from the special approach at Fairley House and have seen our daughter flourish again. She will rejoin the mainstream of schooling in the next academic year and we are both hopeful and apprehensive. Nevertheless, we know what the problems may be and we are far better equipped through understanding to meet them in the future. Our main regret is that it took so long to identify dyslexia and start to deal with it. The frustration that our daughter must have suffered is hard to imagine and regrettably not all the scars can heal.

Joe's mother

With one of my sons who had more difficulties than the others, we embarked on a time-consuming and tiring regime where we chose to seek different teachers – a speech therapist, an occupational therapist and someone to help pull the strands together towards carrying out his school work. At this time many miles were covered and there were hours of waiting which had an impact on my time available for the other children in the family. This inevitably meant less time for each and resentment, with its ensuing behaviour and emotional upheaval.

Ian's mother

Ian lacks self-confidence, since he feels he has failed in so many things. He hates reading and most evenings, at homework time, we have a shouting and screaming match between mother and son, because he does not want to read. 'I hate reading, reading's boring.' This is his normal everyday comment. A similar pattern follows with maths. These scenes obviously allow a tense atmos-phere to arise at homework time, which we all dread! My patience runs dry and this makes it difficult for me to help my other two children with their homework.

David's mother

The anxiety and stress associated with having a child with learning difficulties has taken its toll on my own well-being and that of my husband. Tempers have often been short. One of the most taxing factors is not ever being able to take things for granted: that instruc-tions will be carried out; that he will perceive a situation in the way we do; complete a job properly; remember, etc. In short he requires a lot of subtle supervision. For David, his difficulties have been an enormous burden. At times it has made him very miserable and combative and he so wants not to be different.

Rebecca's father

Our daughter had been happy in school up to the time when her lessons took on a more serious form. Her perfect behaviour in school was in complete contrast to the awkward, difficult and unhappy child she was developing into at home. She tried to hide within the class because her school books were empty and the teachers ignored her because she was not disruptive. She fought against going to school every morning.

My wife was the first to realize that our daughter was one of the class's late readers. She spent several hours every day with her one summer holiday teaching her how to read. Our daughter, although very resistant, took the rudiments of learning from my wife. The emotional stress both parties suffered took many months to fade away. What had become clear from this experience was that our daughter could not retain certain information no matter how often she went over it.

I experienced the same problems in teaching our daughter her multiplication tables. I used the same method I had previously used with my son. Learning by rote. No matter how often we went over them, there would be a hole in the middle of certain tables, numbers 7, 8 and 9 of various tables could not be grasped. It was absolutely infuriating. A bit like painting the Bristol Suspension Bridge. You start at one end and before you can complete the task you have defects at the beginning or in the middle and you have to go back to the beginning again.

Having learnt to read it soon became apparent that there was a problem with writing. To get her to write anything at all was a major effort and the few lines she did write under duress were indecipherable. She deliberately disguised her writing because she knew she could not spell. Her words contained no vowels!

We raised the matter with our daughter's school and decided to have her independently assessed. The report was made available to the school. However, it did not receive general acceptance. Within her school there were two trains of thought. One, 'She seems a bright pleasant child who clearly has learning difficulties.' The other opinion was expressed to us by no lesser person than the vice headmaster, that she was a pleasant happy little girl who was not very bright and we were pushy parents who could not adjust to the reality of having a not very bright child. We were the parents of a very unhappy, rude, disruptive, untruthful little girl with no self-esteem. Our little girl had two personae, one for home and one for school. She suffered socially and was desperate to make friends. Her best friend at school was warned off being friendly with her because she was a child with a problem and other children seemed to have been made aware of it. We had made the mistake of discussing her situation with a set of parents whom we thought had become our friends as well as their daughter, our daughter's best friend.

Today, three years later, our child is a well-adjusted, happy, confident girl who is a delight at home and who would never tell a lie no matter what the consequences. We are confident that she is moving on to secondary education having won a place in a small school which has recognized her potential and we hope will provide the additional help she may need to realize that potential.

Gary's mother

It has now been three years since Gary was first assessed as a child with severe ADD (Attention Deficit Disorder) coupled with specific learning difficulties. His difficulties have affected me deeply, as if by process of osmosis his frustration resulting from his dyslexia had become my source of anxiety and frustration. The ADD traits have presented an inexhaustible amount of stress in everyday life. The often demanding nature of an ADD child, together with his inability to rationalize a situation, is an aspect of life that parents of these children have to live with. I feel that the families of these children need extra help to give them guidance and confidence in dealing with these very demanding children.

I began to think I was being judged as an incompetent parent, because my child's behaviour was often unreasonable or inappropriate. This negative opinion must have generated a sense of low self-esteem which would naturally have been conveyed to Gary. I am sure that I had become oversensitive in my reaction and response to the situation.

It was not until I learned that Gary's problems are largely due to his neurological condition that I began to believe that I was not doing everything wrong to cause those tantrums and persistent demands that he made. Until I learned to accept him as a whole with his difficulties being part and parcel of his personality, I was in essence the one with a problem. Consequently, all attempts to find an alternative 'cure', which in the years have included cranial osteopathy, acupuncture, physiotherapy, vitamin supplementary diet, etc., have now been abandoned. Instead of trying to rid Gary of his ADD, he has recently been placed on medication to help him cope with ADD and this has so far proven successful. Giving Gary this medication is the acceptance of his condition and not rejecting it as indicated by the previously relentless efforts to find a magical end to the problem. I am sure Gary too feels relieved that we have stopped our quest for the Holy Grail, as he no longer has to put up the fights of protest whenever he was taken to a therapist of one sort or another. The proof is that when asked how differently he felt on medication he thought about it for a moment and said, 'I feel like I want to be helpful'.

John's father

The more we have learned about the 'problem' the clearer it is that much more could and should be done, as a matter of course, to diagnose learning problems in mainstream schools at an early stage and to provide appropriate help. The evidence for the 'cost-effectiveness' of such a change is overwhelming.

Jack's mother

As soon as Jack was diagnosed as an 'at risk' dyslexic when he was four and a half, we were able to begin explaining to him that he might find it more difficult than most to learn how to read and write. It was only when Jack made the deliberate and absolute decision to deprive himself of his nightly story that I realized he had consciously obliterated the idea that words could bring pleasure; for him, they brought pressure and punishment. But he knew he needed them and therein also lay pain.

You may not choose to print this, but goodness, what a wonderfully cathartic exercise.

The parents, like their children, responded to the task of describing what dyslexia meant to them with frankness, perception and often emotion, as is evident from the views above. It must be remembered, however, that these are the parents who have found substantial support for their children. There are many more who are still struggling to make sense of their children's difficulties and are watching them fail for lack of appropriate help.

Selection for specialist intervention

Applicants for a school like Fairley House, where dyslexic children are offered an intensive remedial programme for a limited period of time (usually two to three years), present different problems at different ages. The prognosis for each individual will vary. The factors in common are the marked discrepancy between the child's potential and their performance in all or any of the areas of reading, writing, spelling and arithmetic and the fact that this discrepancy is the consequence of specific learning difficulties. Severe visual or auditory impairment, emotional or behavioural difficulties, physical handicap, low ability level or incomplete mastery of the English language can all be prime factors in adversely affecting a child's academic career. They may compound the problem of the dyslexic child. However, if they are the prime cause of school failure, a period of total immersion in a school specifically designed for dyslexic children is unlikely to be the right solution.

The expertise of the multidisciplinary team at Fairley House, which includes an Educational Psychologist, Speech and Language and Occupational Therapists, specialist remedial teachers and classteachers qualified to teach children with specific learning difficulties, is focused on the dyslexic aspects of the child's performance. Children would not be accepted whose problems in one specific area were so profound that they could not access even a modified curriculum in the classroom or who would require daily individual sessions with the Speech and Language or Occupational Therapist, since a balance of provision must be established for all children, who all need their share of time and attention.

One of the commonest reasons for declining to accept a child is the realization that more or better targeted support within the mainstream system would be adequate. To accept these children would be 'taking a sledgehammer to crack a nut'. They would also use up places needed for children whose problems are proving so extensive and persistent that continuation in the mainstream system is unrealistic and could even prove damaging.

There are two areas where symptoms often overlap and boundaries are hard to establish between dyslexia and other syndromes. The first is evident when a child has attention deficit hyperactive disorder (ADHD), which is not uncommonly present in dyslexic children but can be diagnosed as a distinct problem in its own right. It certainly inhibits learning and requires careful management. In extreme cases these children will distract not only themselves, but also classteachers and peers to such an extent that there is constant disruption in lessons. Should this seem probable, caution is exercised in accepting the child. At the very least such children would be brought into the school for a day or two before being offered a place. An experienced classteacher could then comment on whether the degree of hyperactivity precluded consistent attention to tasks or the successful interaction and communication with staff and other pupils. The Headteacher and the Educational Psychologist would then take the final decision and, if the child was not accepted, would advise on an alternative placement.

The second area of concern, which emerges more rarely but can impede progress to a significant extent, centres around affective disorders and various degrees and types of depression. Jonathan Cohen (1994) writes:

> It is important that parents, educators and health care providers be attuned to the signs and symptoms of depression in childhood and understand how it may be related to attentional, reading and other learning problems.

His article entitled 'On the differentional diagnosis of reading, attentional and depressive disorders' sets out clearly how problems in any of these areas interact with and compound each other.

Diagnosis of either ADHD or depression in children is complex and there are important implications for educational management. It is beyond the scope of those in the teaching profession to identify or analyse the presence of ADHD or depressive disorders without referring to the Educational Psychologist, Neurologist or Paediatrician for expert advice. However, unless there is general recognition in schools of some of the presenting symptoms, referral may not be made and inappropriate management may exacerbate the learning difficulties of the individual child concerned. The child or the whole family may need therapeutic counselling before the pupil can benefit fully from the intensive remedial programme which is on offer.

The needs of the children who are accepted are diverse enough to require individual educational programmes which are clearly defined, closely monitored and constantly revised. Prognosis will reflect variations in attitude, IQ, emotional stability, levels of parental support, age and cultural background. The severity of the dyslexic symptoms does not always determine the expected rate of progress, which can be unpredictable. Initial prognosis must always be cautious.

In order to establish whether children will be suitable candidates for a period of total immersion in a specialist school, full and detailed assessment on site is essential. The Educational Psychologist, Speech and Language Therapist, Occupational Therapist and Headteacher will make their own individual diagnoses and establish from their own perspectives whether the intensive remedial programmes offered would be effective.

The multidisciplinary assessment team defines the barriers to learning, each in their own area, and the management of each individual pupil will be based on their reports and comments. Much time will be saved because, from the beginning, a holistic view of the child will have been obtained. Although theory is important and all the members of the team will be aware of research developments in the field and of the concept and definitions of dyslexia, there is no substitute for the practical experience gained by working as a team, on site, for a continuing period. At the case conference following an assessment, it is very rare for the professional team to disagree as to the suitability of a candidate or the nature of their difficulties.

Summary

In the following chapters representatives of several professional disciplines will approach the whole subject of dyslexia from their different perspectives. No one clear definition will emerge, but certain patterns will become apparent. Careful diagnosis of the presenting symptoms results in clear implications for effective management. It is only through the crossfertilization of ideas, through ongoing communications between the professionals and cooperation at every stage between all those involved with the child, including the parents, that successful remedial strategies can be evolved.

References

Cohen, J. (1994) On the differential diagnosis of reading, attentional and depressive disorders. *Annals of Dyslexia, an Interdisciplinary Journal of the Orton Dyslexia Society*, **XLIV**, 165–84.

Hinshelwood, J. (1917) *Congenital Word-Blindness*, H.K. Lewis, London.

Miles, E. (1995) Can there be a single definition of dyslexia? *Journal of the British Dyslexia Association*, **1**(1), 37–44.

Orton, S.T. (1937) *Reading, Writing and Speech Problems in Children*, W.W. Norton, New York.

Rawson, M. (1995) *Dyslexia over a Lifespan*, Educators Publishing Service Inc., Cambridge, Mass.

Further reading

Augur, J. Information on Dyslexia for Schools. British Dylsexia Association Leaflet, Reading.

Carlisle, J. (1995) Dyslexia: A Guide for the Medical Profession. British Dyslexia Association Leaflet, Reading.

Miles, T. (1993) *Dyslexia: The Pattern of Difficulties*, 2nd edn, Whurr, London.

Pumfrey, P. and Reason, R. (1991) *Specific Learning Difficulties (Dyslexia): Challenges and Responses*, NFER Routledge, London.

Snowling, M. (1987) *Dyslexia: A Cognitive Development Perspective*, Blackwell, Oxford.

Thomson, M. (1990) *Developmental Dyslexia: The Nature, Assessment and Remediation*, 3rd edn, Whurr, London.
Vellutino, F. (1979) *Dyslexia Theory and Research*, MIT Press, Cambridge, Mass.

Useful sources of information

British Dyslexia Association
98 London Road
Reading RG1 5AU

Dyslexia Computer Resource Centre
Department of Psychology
Hull University
Hull HU6 7RX

Dyslexia Institute
133 Gresham Road
Staines TW18 2AJ

2 *The Educational Psychologist*

Peter Gilchrist

David

The piece of written work in Fig. 2.1 was produced by a boy who, as yet, had not been diagnosed as having a specific learning disability.

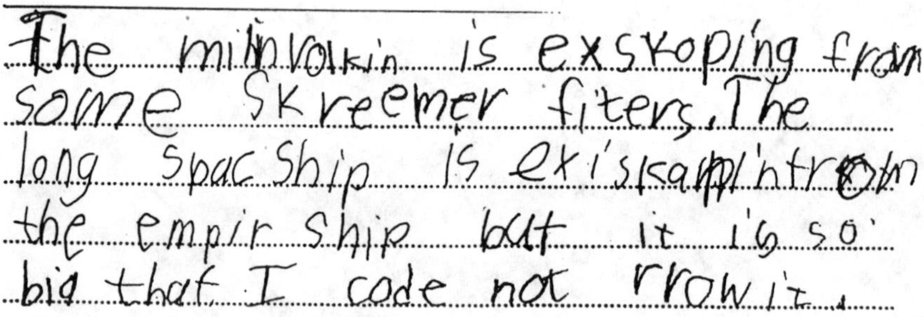

The milnvolkin is exsroping from some skreemer fiters. The long spac ship is exi'ssampi'htrom the empir ship but it i'g so' big that I code not rrow it.

Fig. 2.1 Produced by David aged 9½.

David was 9½ years of age and seemed relatively bright in his early days, but was now becoming increasingly negative and lacking in confidence. He was even turning up late for training for his beloved football team and had been dropped from the first eleven as a result.

At a summer parent–teacher meeting the Headmaster asked if he might have a word with David's parents, who were already becoming increasingly concerned about their son's performance and general happiness. They were now even more alarmed to be summoned to the Head's office, where they were given a cup of tea and invited to make themselves comfortable while the Head mused over some of his papers.

'Mr and Mrs Jones, we really must do something about David. He really is becoming very distractible and, at times, rather disruptive in class. Teachers are finding him irritating, difficult to manage and he is disrupting the work of those around him.'

Having pushed two or three of David's exercise books across the desk to the boy's parents, he continued, 'He really is making so little effort with his work – this is as much as we seem to be able to get out of him at present. May I suggest that we ask our Educational Psychologist if he would have a look at David to advise us how best to proceed'.

It will come as no surprise to discover that David proved to be dyslexic.

The Psychologist's role in the diagnosis of dyslexia

Before beginning the search for an effective diagnosis and treatment for dyslexia, or specific learning disabilities, we need to look very carefully at the criteria on which such a diagnosis is based. There are so many myths, old wives' tales and misunderstandings associated with dyslexia that it is crucial that we know the background from which we speak. Indeed, it is fair to say that there is a considerable lobby that considers that dyslexia simply does not exist and is a figment of the middle-class urge to explain children's academic frailties rather than accept laziness or the almost intolerable prospect of inadequate ability.

First and foremost, dyslexia is a deficit of information processing. We all spend every waking moment of our lives processing a wide variety of visual, auditory, olfactory and kinaesthetic sensory inputs. Some of these are processed quite unconsciously and others reach our conscious awareness and become the apparent criteria upon which we make decisions and alter our behaviour.

For example, if you were to find yourself standing on a busy Underground station with a train roaring through the tunnel towards your platform, there are a number of different types of information to be processed rapidly if you are to find a place on a rush-hour tube. It is equally important, of course, to protect personal safety and not be pushed under the rapidly approaching train. The time, the train's destination and the level of crowding are all very conscious criteria, whereas spatial concepts and the judgement of the speed, for example, are virtually unconscious but may be equally crucial in making a sound decision.

I only mention this practical, everyday example of sensory information processing to make it quite clear that we are not necessarily discussing purely language-related information, much less simply reading and spelling. For example, the impulsiveness of the dyslexic is well described in the literature. A significant number of dyslexics will launch themselves into a social situation without processing enough of the available information and as a result their advances meet with a rebuff or their comments seem bewilderingly inappropriate. This is especially true where dyslexia is exacerbated by an attention deficit, which magnifies the distractible impulsiveness considerably.

Language-related information processing

If we look a little more specifically at dyslexics and their capacity to process spoken language, we find a statistically significant tendency to be muddled by complex incoming language. They often confuse instructions in class, simple directions or details of how a game should be played, for example. Once again the child so often looks muddled, responds inappropriately and far too often attempts to comply are rejected and the child is left feeling stupid, with morale crushed. The deflating and demoralizing impact of specific learning disabilities simply cannot be overstated.

Secondly, the same individuals, having eventually understood exactly what is required, may be equally confused and immature in their capacity to express their own meaning. Frequently in their early development there is a history of poor rhyming skills. Considerable work will have to be undertaken with these children to help them deal with their ability to think and organize language and to produce effective spoken responses before it makes sense to embark on the symbolic language of reading and writing.

A basic truth surrounding the dyslexic phenomenon suggests that each individual is so dramatically different from the last that children with specific learning difficulties are almost a non-homogeneous group. There is a spectrum of symptoms associated with dyslexia and seldom do all exist, at a profound level, in a single individual. Clearly, this makes the work of the teacher in class very complex, as we will hear later in the book, as the symptoms and eccentricities of each child in the group will have to be borne very carefully in mind. The teacher will find one child processes spoken language perfectly adequately, while another does not; with another fine motor skills are appalling and need a great deal of help and yet a third actually manages at a perfectly competent, average level. Why does David read well when he simply cannot spell, for example?

Finally, we move towards the very much more recognizable world of dyslexia – the manipulation and processing of letter symbols. Early on in a child's school life or later in the life of the very disabled dyslexic child, the principal concern revolves around the decoding of very simple letter symbols in the form of single-syllable words, in very short sentences. For some children, even this first step into literacy becomes a bewildering minefield of complexity, in which letter and word shapes mean little and are all too easily forgotten and in which the significance of the direction and sequence of letters means next to nothing. For these children an awareness that words can be broken down into their letter sounds, or phonic components, and the knowledge that there is usually a letter symbol or combination of symbols associated with each sound can become a haven of understanding of the decoding process. However, this phonological process can prove disturbingly elusive.

In essence, reading is simply the decoding of symbolic language, produced, usually, by somebody else. It is a code that allows us to communicate with people whom we may never meet. It is a marvellous, sophisticated medium for the transmission of ideas, stories, poetry – indeed, an 'Aladdin's Cave' of language. For some this code is desperately difficult to break.

The encoding process of producing written information is more complex still. It is, of course, processed rather differently in the brain and involves skills and sensory inputs not required for reading. This explains the typical dyslexic gulf that so often occurs between comparatively competent reading and disabled spelling and written work. There will often be a three or four year gap between these two skills. With little or no phonic skills, poor visual memory and very awkward fine motor skills which make the coordination of a pen so difficult, the wonder is that youngsters ever communicate in written form at all.

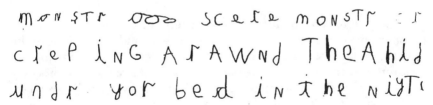

Fig. 2.2 Classic example of dyslexic writing.

In Fig. 2.2, we have the most obvious and clearcut manifestation of dyslexia. This young man's work produced classic examples of letter reversals, bizarre, inappropriate spellings, very awkward letter formation and disjointed, rather staccato written expression as a whole.

The hidden information-processing deficit

Unfortunately for dyslexic sufferers, their disability extends so much further than the mechanical interpretation or production of letter symbols in word-making combinations. It also affects the processing of the underlying information contained in these words, sentences, paragraphs and chapters. This tends to be especially true of the youngster whose reading has made rapid and dramatic progress. Often it is found that their visual scanning of the material and apparent fluency mask a total inability to process the content of the passage. One can well imagine the dramatic effect that this difficulty will have on the older, brighter dyslexic, who is attempting to cope with the rigours of examinations.

The confusion often extends into the planning and organization of creative writing. It is so typical to find a bright youngster of ten years of age producing an essay describing 'my favourite holiday', only to find the family actually reaching Devon in the last paragraph!

In essence, dyslexia concerns itself principally with information processing associated with the organization of language and, especially, symbolic language. Initial remedial input may be aimed at grasping the mysteries of letter symbols and their organization, whether this be in reading or spelling. However, we must look still further at an individual's capacity to comprehend and access or, indeed, communicate the information underlying these symbols. Mechanical reading that means nothing to the reader and chaotically disorganized written information that fails to communicate are both frustratingly worthless endeavours.

Preschool disposing factors

Having established our fundamental criteria of dyslexia, it is already becoming increasingly apparent that while each individual is very different from the last, we have begun to focus attention on an identifiable syndrome. We accept that a breakdown in a child's capacity to process a wide variety of different types of information may well predispose them to dyslexia. Very early evidence may exist which suggests areas of vulnerability in information processing which predispose the child to what we describe as dyslexia.

Paula Tallal (1995) has described the fact that very young infants can be taught to respond to an auditory signal. There appears to be an immense difference between some children who can detect a signal of only 50 or 60 milliseconds in duration, while others only respond to a 300-millisecond signal. It is suggested that more mature dyslexics have a similar pattern in their capacity to respond to auditory signals. If the speed and ease with which we can respond to language and language-related signals are very important functions in literacy acquisition, in time we may be able to isolate the vulnerable and at-risk child at a remarkably early stage in their development.

There are already a number of researchers (Bradley, 1988; Snowling *et al.*, 1986; Tallal, 1980) who have looked at the early development of language, not only the development of literacy skills, but the broader significance of inadequate language development in itself. Hence, late development of language may well be one of our earliest pointers to vulnerability.

Experience over the past 15 years at Fairley House has suggested that the majority of children who present for assessment have experienced early difficulties with language acquisition. This includes late-developing language per se, otitis media necessitating the fitting of grommet tubes, difficulties of articulation and/or a tendency to confuse the naming of objects in their environment, which often leads to the mispronunciation of names or even a frantic search for appropriate labels in the first place, together with grammatical and syntactical inaccuracies in the way in which language is processed. A history of this type occurs far less often in the population at large.

As the essence of dyslexia revolves around inadequate language-related information processing, we can see what an early stumbling block this would prove to be. These children find auditory processing extremely difficult. The early language models laid down as they acquire speech are inaccurate and imprecise but form the basis on which their phonic attack is founded, with the predictable inaccuracies and confusions that one might anticipate.

Early mobility and gross and fine motor skills also form an important basis for education. A child's ability to perceive their position in space, either moving among friends or sitting appropriately at a desk, is in itself important. Even more so is the capacity to organize the child's body at a desk and to manipulate the writing hand in the formation of letters and words. So often, one of the greatest frustrations for a bright, dyslexic child revolves around a tremendous grasp of language and thought processes, possibly even excellent reading, and a total incapacity to produce effective written language. Much of this weakness finds its root in poor fine motor skills.

While in research and in associations with understandable vested interests in a particular disability, there is an urge to keep syndromes separate, in reality this is quite impossible. Hence, attention deficit disorder (ADD) is an important overlapping factor for a small but nevertheless significant number of our dyslexic children. The child who simply cannot sit still, is unable to stay on task for more than a few seconds, is constantly disruptive and, ultimately, rather rejected and alienated from their peer group is hardly predisposed to effective early learning. So often these young people are simply 'unavailable for learning' and so much of early school experience passes them by, leaving them trailing in the wake of peers of similar ability, partly because their attention deficit has undermined their capacity to focus their attention. Where this problem is compounded by dyslexic vulnerabilities, the prognosis is certainly not improved and early diagnosis and treatment become even more crucial.

Another early sign may revolve around the irritating and frustrating inability to organize the child's belongings, cope with time or even remember where they should be next. Considering the complexity of processing information, even for a child to move from one part of a nursery class to begin a different task, possibly in cooperation with another child, it is much easier to understand that if these activities are not processed in perfect synchrony, confusion and distress may ensue. The individual involved may feel angry and resentful that other people seem able to cope so easily and yet they are having to look at their neighbours' behaviour even to follow comparatively simple instructions.

At the very top end of nursery school, when some children are beginning to develop the early stages of reading and writing, we may find a 'tell-tale' gulf already emerging between a child's language skills and an apparent inability to cope with letter symbols.

At home, this is especially true of the child whose problems also include dyspraxia. They often confuse social and domestic information processing, frequently leading to conflict. Early morning, preparing for school, is a classic time of crisis. The same may well be true of homework and bed times. The child departing for school with only one gym shoe, homework still in the bedroom, school tie and shoe laces untied presents such a familiar picture. If these youngsters are to cope in an organized fashion in class, strategies to help their domestic planning will form a crucial part of treatment.

Early school signs

It is a common and worrying precept that there is no need to refer children for investigation or to be unduly concerned about the slow development of literacy before 6½ to 7 years of age. It is certainly true that children develop at different speeds, even those of very similar intellectual capacity, and that some children take considerable time to settle into the routine of school. They must learn, especially those who have no previous preschool experience, how to share and give and take with their peers.

I would certainly not wish to encourage any undue anxiety in parents or stress in children facing the rigours of their first year of school life. However, it is fair to say that the warning signs may well be quite apparent, even in the first or second term of school. Once again, prevention is so much better than cure and prevention of serious learning disabilities will allow for a very much happier and less stressful journey through the early stages of education. We must remember that in so many schools, once a child reaches eight or nine years of age there is less and less accent on reading and literacy acquisition, as it is assumed that these skills are by now available to the child.

We may assume that the first three years of school life are fundamentally concerned with three key targets. First and foremost, a child must learn to adapt to the complexities of a school day, to share with other children and learn that a day has its pattern and cycle and that different activities will be expected at different times of the day. Hence, there will be a time for music, play, art and sport, but at other times, especially during the mornings, the child will be expected to sit still for increasing periods of time and concentrate on tasks, some of which will challenge new boundaries but others, which may appear to be boringly repetitive, will be consolidating half-developed ground.

Much of this territory will be covered in Chapter 9 by Angela Dominy and Nicholas Rees, who have considerable experience in dealing with children with specific learning disabilities. Nevertheless, from a psychologist's point of view, there are several hallmarks of possible concern which parents, teachers and psychologists would wish to address.

The classic presenting symptoms of a specific learning disability is the child who, before break, appears an articulate, responsive and almost dominant contributor within their discussion group. Yet this same child, on return after break, when asked to produce a **written** response, alters position in the 'pecking order' as they struggle to cope. They seem much less able than they appeared only minutes earlier.

We are all aware of children who, for no apparent reason, seem to find reading a desperately difficult task. Words confronted and rehearsed on one page appear totally forgotten on the next. They learn spelling lists one evening and seem to be relatively competent and, indeed, may produce an adequate score the following morning, but residual memory, seven days later, is only marginal. This constant peaking and troughing of the learning curve becomes discouraging, depressing and demotivating. It is so very difficult for a parent or even a teacher not to assume that in some way this behaviour is wilful or that with greater effort and a more profound level of concentration, all would be well and the child would be quite capable of remembering.

Hence, we are confronting the first and possibly most telling symptom of dyslexia – poor short-term memory function. In the very early days, visual memory will be crucial, when a child is learning to copy a line of the teacher's writing; flash cards, 'look and say' and the acquisition of a sight vocabulary will be essential ingredients of literacy development. The problems that poor visual memory for symbols can cause are only too apparent (Benton, 1974; Miles, 1993).

We referred to poor fine motor skills during the preschool days and these will now become a particular hazard during the first two or three years of formal schooling. If a child seems to find copying simple shapes or manipulating a fine point like a pencil extremely difficult, then a gap will begin to emerge very rapidly between language skills, reading and a capacity to produce written work. It may well be that as they move through their second school year, written work will still be brief, untidy and poorly executed for a child who seems, in so many other ways, to be of reasonable ability.

Inadequate language development, so familiar in the dyslexic child, is perhaps the most worrying facet of early school life as it can so easily mask underlying ability (Frith, 1985). There are, after all, comparatively few signals which allow anyone to judge the ability of a child. We look at the ability to integrate and relate socially; the quality of work produced compared with a child's peers; and, above all, the way in which spoken language skills are used. If children's written work is immature, they seem to find relationships very difficult and their language is much less mature than those around them, the assumption can often be that they are of limited ability.

Low ability may, of course, be the case; 16–18% of children in the general population have IQs below 85. However, what of the youngster with poor fine motor skills and a major language-processing disability, but with an IQ above 120? We have worked time and again with children who produce remarkable test scores, often in the superior range, and yet become very muddled by complex language input and equally confused in making their own meaning clear. Poor fine motor coordination and inadequate letter formation are also common in dyslexic children and in the dyspraxic youngster, whose disabilities often overlap with those of the dyslexic. (Ingrid Linge discusses dyspraxia at length in Chapter 4.)

Attention deficit disorder (with or without hyperactivity), referred to earlier, can also be a contributing factor. Poor concentration will tend to magnify learning difficulties. As the academic demands increase, especially in the second and third years of school life, so difficulties of selective attention will become not only increasingly manifest, but more irritating to the children themselves and to those attempting to teach them.

Dr Sam Tucker discusses the management of attention deficit disorder in Chapter 6. It is difficult to imagine how irritating it must be for the individual to find that a span of concentration lasts for little more than 20–30 seconds, before sights and sounds around become as absorbing as the task in hand. This is particularly evident in consolidation work in class, where arousal level is not especially high in the child. Frustratingly, once their interest level and arousal rise beyond a certain threshold, their problems become very much less apparent. However, nobody can remain in 'overdrive' all day long (Barkley, 1990). At home, the child may well be becoming increasingly disenchanted with school. Headaches, tummy aches, bed wetting, tears before school, increasing conflict with siblings, not to mention somewhat turbulent and emotional outbursts in the hour or so after returning from school, are all familiar in the history of dyslexic children. This behaviour is far from easy to manage but we must remember how frustrating it is to find that what appears to be second nature to others, who may well be perceived as being less able, is extremely difficult for the dyslexic child.

Mid-school – 8–12 years old

The early school factors are now becoming more ingrained and attitudes are hardening, both in teachers and parents who by now may well perceive their child as lazy, obstinate, difficult and unpredictable.

If we recall the example of David and the meeting of his anxious and troubled parents with the Headteacher, we are forced to accept, yet again, that an understanding of the condition remains worryingly superficial. However, to be entirely fair to both parents and teachers, the dyslexia can be the 'great chameleon' in that a child with any spirit may well mask deficiencies with a variety of attention-seeking ploys. As far as work is concerned it is often far easier for the ego, even at a subconscious level, to allow the world to imagine that so much more could be achieved if the effort were made. It is much more difficult to accept inadequacy as part of a self-image. Hence, a poor attitude and behaviour problems often emerge at this stage in the child's life, when the world is becoming much more demanding and critical.

The gulf between ability and the youngster's reading and, more particularly, spelling and written work is likely to be more clearly established. However, it is not unusual in these years to find a child whose reading seems relatively fluent, although their comprehension is extraordinarily faulty. Especially in the centre of a passage, where the text is at its densest, a child may readily revert to the exercise of analysing each word, struggling to scan evenly from left to right, rather than processing reading as a form of language. The smaller the print, the more problems there are likely to be. This is especially true of the child to whom reading came late in their development and for whom the activity may eventually have developed very rapidly. It is important to be absolutely sure that the child is, in fact, extracting information from the text.

The area of literacy development which will almost certainly be seriously affected is the processing of written language. Spelling is an important part of this process but the organization of ideas, themes and images into written language is often extremely difficult for the dyslexic child. There is an understandable tendency to cling to simple vocabulary which can readily be spelt, rather than using the very much richer vocabulary apparently available to the child. Furthermore, slow fine motor coordination makes letter formation difficult and tiring and the actual mechanics of writing tend to overwhelm the processing of ideas. Once again, we are confronted with dyslexia as a deficit in information processing (Snowling, Stackhouse and Rack, 1986).

Obviously, if children can neither process incoming language adequately nor organize thoughts and spoken language effectively, it is unrealistic to expect them to do any better with their written work. Jeanne Reilly, in her chapter on the work of the Speech and Language Therapist, has pursued these issues at greater length.

At the top end of this age group, especially in the private sector of education, sophisticated processing of written information becomes a particular burden and a crucial remedial target. This is particularly true once examinations of any importance appear on the horizon. Very few dyslexic children, and even fewer with a dyspraxic overlay, know how to set about effective study. Revision and notetaking are bewildering mysteries to this group, as is the devising of anything resembling a revision schedule. More worryingly, children with specific learning disabilities typically fall into two major traps when asked to process sophisticated information under pressure, as in examinations. Firstly, they misinterpret the longer, wordier examination questions, producing apparently adequate answers which are far from relevant, or they simply panic at the sight of a lengthy question and 'snatch' at three or four key words, inventing their own version. In both such eventualities their success will depend largely on luck.

Secondly, with their disorganized approach to written language, these children tend to overwrite, leaving exam papers unfinished or, possibly even worse, finishing with a great deal of time to spare, which must imply that their answers are too superficial. These problems are magnified still further for the children with poor fine motor skills, who have to write slowly if they are to retain legibility and, therefore, brevity is forced upon them.

For the young person with a serious degree of fine motor difficulty the touch-typing programme, which is dealt with by Patience Thomson in Chapter 8, has opened a fascinating 'window' onto a whole new level of written communication for these children. After the initial and not inconsiderable hurdle of learning to touch type, usually achieved in the space of a single term, the youngster rapidly becomes much swifter, always legible and, of course, has access to a spell check and thesaurus. Benefits later in the education process, particularly in projects, coursework and examinations, prove immeasurable.

Adolescent and young adult criteria

Many of the factors discussed at the end of the last section are equally true for the adolescent. We are now beginning to see a significant number of the early Fairley House students reaching maturity and public examinations. Information-processing difficulties are an almost universal problem for this group but, once dealt with, they have achieved a remarkable degree of success and have often proceeded on to university education in due course. I feel sure that they would be the first to agree that without considerable help on their study skills and exam technique, this success would have been denied them.

If we return yet again to dyslexia as a function of inadequate information processing, we must look at its impact long after the child has learned to read and spell competently. We cannot assume that the deficits which impeded the development of early literacy have, in some mysterious way, vanished. For example, when the 18-year-old dyslexic is being assessed for a certificate requesting extra time in examinations, confused, slow and inaccurate information processing is often the basis for these arrangements and not a deficit in spelling per se. Some of them are, of course, appalling spellers and an allowance can readily be made for this. However, it is a much less important therapeutic target, at this stage in a child's education, than study skills and exam technique.

For the undiagnosed and untreated dyslexic, this may well be the most worrying phase of their development. It is hardly any wonder if such a child finds school attendance a far from attractive prospect. Why keep confronting an environment in which life is usually unsuccessful and where there is a constant 'loss of face' among peers who seem so easy to dominate in other facets of life?

Imagine the stress created by waking every morning to know that failure is inevitable yet again. Each of us has a different way of dealing with this type of stress. Becoming depressed, tearful, withdrawn, angry and avoiding social contact in school, including poor school attendance, are all very understandable responses, often totally misinterpreted both at home and in school. Frustration, bouts of aggression, wilful and rather unpredictable behaviour are also hardly surprising.

We must also look at the tendency to find other ways of bolstering a somewhat battered ego and diminished self-image. A drift towards mischief, whether this be petty theft, alcohol or drug abuse, or truanting, may well depend on the individual's social contacts and family mores. Sadly, however, it is not unusual to find children drifting from the 'straight and narrow', even in the most supportive families. With caring parents, the feeling of failure and having disappointed those who matter most may be even more painful.

In essence, one of the tell-tale signs of a specific learning disability which may never have been diagnosed in the adolescent will be the gulf between evident ability in so many other ways and brief, untidy and totally disorganized written work. Equally, beware the reports that constantly echo, 'He or she has tried so hard and so consistently throughout the term. What a shame about the exam results'.

The search for a diagnosis

At the outset of our quest into the realms of dyslexia and an exploration of the way in which youngsters process information and, indeed, perceive the world about them, it is vital that the psychologist is well armed with a battery of initial information. Far too often the process is regarded as being almost on a par with 'reading the tea leaves' and that, therefore, prior information, access to previous reports or, indeed, any other preliminary understanding of the child concerned might in some way distort the findings.

It is crucial that we all regard ourselves as part of a team attempting to reassemble a complex jigsaw puzzle, each of us having a clear, distinct and vital role to play in this process.

Long before a psychological assessment takes place, shortly following that preliminary anxious phone call to set an appointment date, a family questionnaire is dispatched to the child's parents. This may often seem like a cross between adult homework and a penance for producing a dyslexic child. However, its true purpose is to give us advance understanding of the child's early developmental history, especially their language development and early mobility. Ear, nose and throat difficulties, often in the preschool years, can be very significant in a child's auditory processing. A family history of specific learning disabilities suggests a hereditary factor and, of course, a brief outline of school history to date, with the problems that the child has been experiencing, provides useful clues. Finally, a 'thumbnail sketch' is helpful, describing exactly how the child's parents perceive the problem about which they seek information and understanding. Patience Thomson has dealt in greater detail with this questionnaire and its purpose but suffice it to say that, from a psychologist's point of view, it gives us our fundamental starting point. There are often reports available following previous investigations by other Educational Psychologists, Speech and Language Therapists, Occupational Therapists, a variety of medical specialities, Orthoptists and, even more frequently, the remedial teachers who have begun the struggle.

Current school reports are also invaluable and earlier ones must not be forgotten as they elucidate the developing pattern over a period of terms and sometimes even years. Furthermore, they not only give us a clear indication of the problems as perceived by the school, especially the class teacher, but also to what extent the underlying dyslexic phenomena have been recognized and are being treated.

Test scores, statistics, numbers – all have their purpose but nothing quite takes the place of typical examples of the work that children are currently attempting. These will demonstrate levels of success, the way the child uses written language, coordinates the use of a pen, organizes work on the page and understands the concepts under discussion, quite apart from the spelling errors which frequently occur. If we add to this a photocopy of a page or two of the reader which the child is currently working on, together with a page of current mathematics, we are able to create a much clearer image of exactly how the youngster is coping within the peer group, against which we can make assumptions based on the norms that apply to this particular age group, given its particular academic environment.

We now need to know a great deal more about the specific individual. The chapters by Ingrid Linge, the school's Occupational Therapist, and Jeanne Reilly, the Speech and Language Therapist, give detailed accounts of their diagnostic and therapeutic input.

Patience Thomson involves the children in a rather more relaxed and often fascinatingly revealing session that she always includes in the assessment profile of the youngsters who visit Fairley House. It is also important to remember the significance of an assessment session in the mind of a small child. It is so easy to assume that this is an experience taken easily in the child's stride when, in reality, failure may have been accumulating steadily over the years. This leads to concern increasingly expressed by both parents and teachers and a huge build-up of stress and anxiety in the child. In reality it is an extraordinary mark of the resilience of young people that the vast majority settle very quickly into their assessment session and actually thoroughly enjoy the experience.

However, it is vital from the psychologist's point of view that nothing of any seriousness is undertaken until the child is put at ease. How possible this proves to be is one of the 'soft signs' that I will discuss a little later in the chapter and to which reference will be made in the written report which is the eventual result of the assessment. A small number of the youngsters remain rather tense and anxious throughout and this necessitates constant breaks from the tests to allow discussion of the world around them until they are comfortable once again. It is crucial to remember that we are assessing a child's capacity to process a wide variety of different types of information, both verbal and non-verbal, and then comparing the outcome with the norms for a child's age group and, therefore, stress must be minimized.

The test information is obviously extremely helpful in making a diagnosis and prescribing treatment, but it would be wrong to assume that IQ test results are 'writ on tablets of stone'. We are simply describing human experience and the information processing of a comparatively young child. There are so many factors affecting a child's performance, quite apart from his own attitude to the experience. For example, a rather distractible, attention-deficit, dyslexic boy was assessed last summer on a very hot, humid afternoon. There was no doubt that towards the end of the afternoon the combination of the weather, the fact that the child tired as his circadian rhythm drifted, as well as the noise of distant traffic, all affected his performance and this must be allowed for in the discussion following the test results.

THE PSYCHOLOGICAL TEST BATTERY

The hard core of the child's assessment will revolve around the Wechsler Intelligence Scale for Children III (WISC III), which was newly standardized in 1992, with support from a variety of other instruments. We have mentioned earlier the need to assess a variety of different facets of information processing and this is exactly what the WISC achieves.

The child works through 12 different subtests, each aimed at assessing a slightly different facet of their intellectual make-up and capacity to organize and deal with a range of quite different concepts. Each is open ended, starting with very simple material from the age of six and moving on to a considerable level of complexity. This allows children to be assessed over a full ten-year range. The child works until they can effectively achieve no more and this becomes the cut-off point in any particular item. The successes achieved yield what is described as a 'raw score' and this is then related to the child's actual age group, which provides us with the scale score that appears on the eventual report.

Although the verbal scale, performance scale and full-scale IQs were separately standardized and therefore scores should not be regarded as precisely an 'averaging', the scale scores which the child achieves are added together, statistics are applied and this then generates an IQ or intelligence quotient.

THE SCATTER OF SUBTESTS

This gives us the first and very important piece of understanding of our dyslexic. Although discrepancies are an invariable factor, we clearly need to know, in essence, exactly how bright the child actually is. It is true that a very ordinary score on an apparently crucial subtest will be of profound significance in a very able child, whilst not being worthy of comment in a child of lesser ability for whom this score is in no way at odds with their profile as a whole. The dyslexic profile is, however, never even in its distribution and an IQ will therefore tend to be statistically deflated by the 'patchy' areas of vulnerability which form the essence of our diagnosis. These symptoms and their significance will be looked at in detail later in the chapter.

THE ROLE OF THE EDUCATIONAL PSYCHOLOGIST

We have established in the first part of this chapter many of the criteria which will be apparent to parents, siblings, friends and, of course, class teachers. Some of these symptoms may already have raised questions about a child's literacy acquisition, but others may seem sufficiently removed from dyslexia not to be readily associated with the syndrome.

Long before embarking upon formal psychometric evaluation, the psychologist's role is to draw together these threads, almost like establishing the corner pieces in what will prove to be a complex jigsaw puzzle.

THE FAMILY QUESTIONNAIRE

In Fairley House and in my practice as a whole, we send a family questionnaire to the parents of a child who has been referred, as discussed earlier. This will need to be amplified in consultation with the parents, which usually involves a lengthy meeting between the mother, father and psychologist immediately after the child's test session has been completed.

Firstly, we are looking for the apparent breakdown in a child's capacity to learn. In other words, what has gone so wrong that parents and teachers feel that an evaluation and a possible placement in a specialist school may be necessary? We go back into the early background of the child and look at the family's own history of learning difficulties. In the vast majority of cases, one or other parent is affected by a similar learning disability and frequently one or more of the siblings. Curiously, the involvement of a parent is a far from negative facet of the diagnosis, as it is much easier to understand the struggles of a child having experienced similar difficulties.

EARLY LANGUAGE HISTORY

A preschool history of ear, nose and throat difficulties is a pattern that cannot be disregarded. The impact of these difficulties, especially when hearing and even language acquisition may be affected, can be observed many years later. Where a child's earliest experiences of language are obscured, so that the word sounds they acquire are less than precise, these then become the phonic models on which they base their spelling so many years later.

For example, at the age of eight or nine, a child may well be pronouncing a word like 'ground' perfectly clearly if asked to say it out aloud and yet when the word is internalized, they refer back to that earlier and inaccurate model. Hence, 'g r o w' emerges for 'ground' or, as was the case with a small boy very recently, the word 'knee' is spelled as 'd e e'. One can almost hear the catarrh and adenoids affecting this child's language development at the age of two or three. We have discussed at some length the impact of language processing itself, quite apart from the articulation of language, earlier in this chapter. We need to be very careful that a child's problems are not simply dismissed because articulation is now within tolerable limits, if the underlying processing of language is still inept. So often these youngsters are dismissed from speech therapy when, in reality, they are still finding it extremely difficult to deal with complex incoming language and are desperately muddled when using speech of any complexity themselves. This is the realm of the Speech and Language Therapist.

Dr Sam Tucker has described in Chapter 6 the involvement of the two different hemispheres of the brain in the control of language and, ultimately, reading. There is considerable research evidence to suggest that dyslexics struggle to shift the control of reading from the right hemisphere, which is more analytical, to the left where it becomes a part of language processing. It is only after this switch has been made satisfactorily that the child will begin to read fluently and derive pleasure from the experience. Once a youngster moves up to a class where reading is required for information gathering, this transfer of processing to the left hemisphere becomes crucial to their success.

FINE AND GROSS MOTOR SKILLS

It will be quite apparent already that if a child's fine motor skills are poor, their written work will usually be untidy, brief and very immature, bearing in mind their age and evident ability in other respects. Drawings will often be equally lacking in maturity and often very simplistic. The difficulties may extend into gross motor weaknesses and difficulties of physical organization. These problems are dealt with in depth in Ingrid Linge's chapter on the work of the Occupational Therapist, especially as they affect the dyspraxic young person.

SHORT-TERM MEMORY

Parents, and even the children themselves, will often refer to poor short-term memory – the constantly muddled messages which so often find the child returning with tasks incomplete. They often find spelling lists, multiplication tables and even telling the time extremely difficult to remember. Indeed, the concept of time as it affects the hours of the day, weeks, months and sequential concepts as a whole is often extremely muddled and confused.

Here we must be aware of the complexity of memory function. So often long- and medium-term memory will be perfectly competent. The child will discuss a holiday taken long ago in the most remarkable and colourful detail and yet will find a spelling list quite impossible to learn.

ATTENTION DEFICIT DISORDER

Distractibility and attention deficit disorder may have been masquerading as a 'difficult child' or even an apparently 'gifted' child 'bored by the dreary teaching in school'. Nevertheless, its management and a clear understanding of the syndrome are important, if a child is to be helped and supported through these crucial years.

DYSPRAXIA

The personal chaos of dyslexic and dyspraxic children is painfully familiar. They find the drawing together of the threads necessary for efficient decision making extremely difficult. Hence, time and again, they will leave for school with their homework still on their bedroom table or, on a day when swimming is on the curriculum, trunks will be left in their drawer at home. So often they are late for class, ill equipped and in constant trouble with their teachers as a result. I cannot overemphasize the necessity for helping a dyslexic to organize day-to-day life thoroughly, as a crucial part of therapy, if they are to be expected to organize their work in school appropriately.

THE PATCHY PROFILE OF THE DYSLEXIC

It is this very 'patchiness' of performance that gives us our dyslexic diagnosis. The brain is unable to process different types of information at the same speed or with equal accuracy and clarity and this in itself causes considerable confusion and self-doubt.

We are in no way suggesting that less able children cannot experience dyslexia but, once again, their profile must also show its own pattern of discrepancy. Equally, a potentially very able child of ten, with a reading age of 8½ and a spelling age of 7 and brief, untidy, poorly presented and spelt written work, has a dramatic level of specific learning disability if we are considering a mental age which may well be nearer 12. It is against this statistical criterion that we must judge the level of impact which the dyslexia is producing.

The average IQ in the United Kingdom should be considered as 100, with 68% of the community having IQs falling between 85 and 115. There are then smaller groups of 15–16% lying between 85 and 70 and 115 and 130 and a tiny number of only 1–2% below and above these points (see Fig. 2.3). IQs will vary a little from test to retest and cannot therefore be regarded as absolute, but the pattern of strengths and vulnerabilities provides an essential clinical profile.

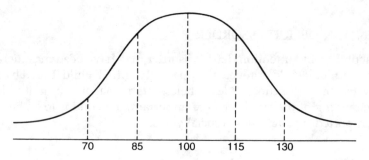

Fig. 2.3 Normal distribution curve of IQ in the UK.

Especially in the private sector of education, it often comes as a considerable surprise to find that many youngsters have IQs falling under 115 and that they actually cope surprisingly well with their academic life. The academic elite with IQs over 125 are comparatively few in number.

However, with an IQ in the average range, dyslexia tends to become a particularly crucial issue, if we look towards public examinations at 16 and 18, especially 'A' levels at the end of their school life. With an IQ of, say, 109, two or even three 'A' levels may prove perfectly possible but this is likely to be severely compromised if the under functioning caused by the specific learning disability is not dealt with robustly.

VERBAL–PERFORMANCE DISCREPANCIES

We have already established that dyslexic individuals do not process information consistently and that this may be apparent at a fundamental level with a large and statistically significant discrepancy between the verbal scale IQ and the performance scale IQ.

For example, Anna has a relatively high verbal scale IQ of 121, with a performance scale IQ of only 98. She has always sounded bright, articulate and knowledgeable about the world around her and yet her work and her literacy skills especially have failed to progress. We now find that it is vulnerabilities on the non-verbal or performance part of her development, looking at practical, spatial, fine motor tasks, visual memory and so forth, that present the greatest difficulty and which have created her specific learning disability.

One of the great myths associated with dyslexia suggests that dyslexics are invariably blessed with a high level of artistic and creative ability. Anna is most certainly not a case in point. Indeed, her diagnosis will have fallen, in large measure, in the province of the Occupational Therapist. Ingrid Linge, in her chapter, will deal with just such an eventuality. In Anna's case we are talking about the overlapping of dyslexia and dyspraxia, which leaves Anna struggling to ensure that her practical and motor activities are effectively accomplished. She has great difficulty with craft, design and technology, for example. In geography when the concept of contour lines was introduced, she was totally bewildered. Indeed, spatial awareness as a whole has always been a great difficulty for this young lady and she even needs to learn how to sit appropriately at her desk, how to hold her pen and how to organize her body in space as a whole. In the creative, practical and spatial world, Anna actually needs additional support.

David, on the other hand, demonstrates a totally different profile. He does not find language easy to process, becomes muddled when instructions are overlengthy and is often not only confused but a little inappropriate in making his meaning clear. In his case, under his comparatively inept language skills lurk very considerable practical, spatial, creative and artistic strengths. The immense difficulty for David is that these abilities have so often gone completely unnoticed and he has begun to feel that he is a complete failure and this will tend to affect any enterprise on which he embarks. Hence, even areas of endeavour which could have been successful are left largely untried. However, properly and sensitively nurtured, this is the group from which we often develop the hugely talented architects of the future, for example.

One of the crucial targets for both teachers and parents of dyslexic youngsters must be the search for strategies for coping with experiences which so many people find comparatively straightforward and yet for the dyslexic prove a stumbling block. This is the point where confidence and an increasing capacity to take risks become so vital in the treatment of dyslexia. With an ambitious search for ways round problems the dyslexic child can eventually become as successful as a peer of similar abilities. With non-verbal strengths, there needs to be a search for success in precisely these areas. The aim should be to harness and develop these talents, as they not only provide a platform of status among a peer group but may well prove the essence of career development later on.

The search for coping strategies is equally essential for the linguistically strong but perceptually disabled children, for whom the use of spoken language must be harnessed as richly as possible, both in terms of subject choice and in the remedial strategies developed in their treatment. For them cassette records and keyboard skills – especially word processing in the later stages of education – may well prove vital survival aids.

Nicholas Rees and Angela Dominy discuss the Fairley House typing programme and its considerable success in Chapter 9.

KEY SUBTESTS

Curiously, some psychologists use only one of these subtests as it is felt that they measure the same linguistic skills. With our dyslexic children this is most certainly not the case. The vocabulary test involves largely a one-word stimulus with a one- or two-word response, the comprehension a lengthy input and complex reply.

Both these subtests reflect cultural influences to a considerable degree. It is almost as though the performance tasks are a measure of the effectiveness of the 'computer' available to the child, while the language or verbal items measure the success of environmental programming. The vocabulary and information subtests are particularly likely to be seriously affected where there is environmental or social and linguistic deprivation, for example. They are also the areas in which family influence has its greatest impact.

However, we have discussed earlier in the chapter the difficulties of language processing which so many of our children experience. Time and again, when a one-word stimulus and a single or two-word response is sufficient the youngster will cope remarkably well, often producing superior scale scores. Once the language input becomes wordy and more complex, children with receptive language problems rapidly become confused as to what is expected of them. Furthermore, if they are also experiencing a poor auditory short-term sequential memory, they may well have forgotten the first part of an instruction whilst struggling to process the last two or three sentences. Should they succeed in organizing the linguistic input satisfactorily, they may still be frustrated, irritated and, at times, even angry by the muddled and inappropriate way in which they organize their own spoken language. It is these very difficulties that are often demonstrated in the comprehension subtest particularly.

The digit span subtest aims at assessing auditory short-term sequential memory, which is a classic area of symptomatic significance in dyslexia. This test requires the child to repeat an increasing number of digits read out by the tester. In the first part repetition is forwards and the children will sometimes adopt a 'chunking' strategy, remembering the numbers in groups. However, when they are requested to repeat them in reverse order this technique proves much more difficult. It is fair to say that with no weakness of short-term memory, either auditory or visual, it is extremely difficult to make a dyslexic diagnosis.

Visual memory is a complex function, much discussed in the literature and still being heavily researched. So much depends on the exact information being processed and the intellectual requirements being made of the child. At Fairley House we use the visual short-term sequential memory subtest from the Illinois Test of Psycholinguistic Ability (ITPA).

The significance of accurate visual memory, particularly of symbols, in early literacy acquisition is quite clear. A weakness in this area continues to have its impact throughout education, especially with far-point copying from blackboards, overhead projectors and even near-point copying from text books. In the early stages sight vocabulary, 'look and say', flashcards and confusion between mathematical symbols are so critically affected.

We also look at laterality in a child's development, by assessing a dominant hand, a dominant foot and eye. It is a fascinating finding that where a child has a right hand and a right foot but a dominant left eye, nine times out of ten they do poorly on the tests of visual memory.

Occasionally, if time permits, the Benton Test of Visual Retention is also used. (For further discussion of visual memory see Ingrid Linge's chapter on perceptual and motor development.)

The coding subtest also involves a degree of visual memory and is often poorly executed in parallel with the Illinois subtest. However, there is also a degree of sequencing involved in this task and, above all, it measures the speed and accuracy with which the child can deal with fine motor coordination. If a dyslexic struggles significantly with this item it is almost certain that their letter formation will be poor and the speed with which they can produce their handwriting desperately slow. Youngsters for whom the processing of written language is the core problem almost all demonstrate this particular vulnerability.

These subtests form the hard core of our dyslexic diagnosis and are at the root of the specific learning disabilities experienced by the vast majority of our children. However, there are one or two other subtests which highlight further particular areas of difficulty. It is often felt that the object assembly and block design reflect similar unusual perceptual and manipulative skills but, once again, dyslexics prove to have their own way of viewing the perceptual world. With the exception of our dyspraxic group, the vast majority of dyslexic children actually function perfectly well and sometimes at a very high level on the block design.

Precisely the same group, on the other hand, may well have great difficulty with the object assembly. Presented with cut-up line drawings which they must reassemble, they find it extraordinarily difficult to perceive in their mind's eye what the finished object should look like and are left hopelessly reliant on random and frequently very frustrated shuffling.

For example, the third of these items is a six-piece cut-up line drawing of a horse (Fig. 2.4), which seems very simple to the non-dyslexic individual and yet to the affected child can become a focus of huge irritation. Time and again, the front legs will emerge from the back of the horse's neck, the body element will appear in what seems to be a giraffe-like neck or truncated horse's body. Certainly, a traditional horse is nowhere to be seen. A subtle form of visual memory, once again, or visual imaging, whose absence is so often part of the dyslexic frustration.

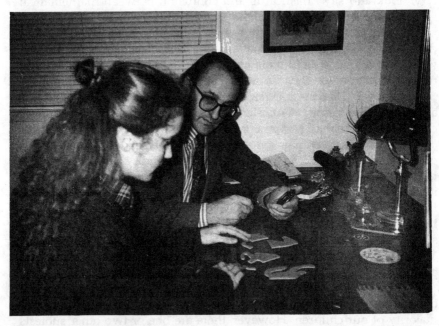

Fig. 2.4 Object assembly.

Finally, on the picture arrangement item children are presented with a series of cartoon strip pictures in random order, which they are asked to sequence appropriately. This task is largely intended to measure visual sequencing skills but our linguistically disadvantaged children often find this task extremely difficult and one must assume that it is the underlying language element in this subtest which is causing so much difficulty. They struggle to see the sequential link between the pictures and tend to become overabsorbed by the content of each card in its own right, rather than searching for a theme. In other words, they struggle to 'tell themselves the story' effectively. It is hardly any wonder if the same child finds essay organization and creative writing almost impossible pursuits.

We may also need to look particularly at the child's mathematical development. In these instances the British Ability Scales Basic Number Skills Test (BAS) is used, which gives us some indication of how effectively a child is dealing with a selection of mathematical concepts, looking firstly at the four basic functions of addition, subtraction, division and multiplication and then moving on to slightly greater sophistication, fractions, decimals and so forth.

SOFT SIGNS

So much of the work of a psychologist is observational and almost intuitive. No statistical justification can be given for soft signs but suffice it to say that they help to understand dyslexics and to paint a clearer picture of their dilemma. Equally, we discussed earlier the complex jigsaw that we struggle to complete and our soft signs certainly contribute.

There are three core issues on which comment should be made in any assessment as they are obviously of vital significance. First and foremost, how well did the child actually relate to the psychologist and were there personal or environmental factors that affected this relationship? Was the youngster at ease and seeming to rather enjoy the experience or did they remain tense and anxious throughout?

Much has been made of language development and processing and this too becomes very apparent at a social and interactional level during the child's session. We are concerned to observe not only how they perform on tests, but to what extent they can make their needs and their feelings known using their language skills. Can they understand and respond to the chat and discussion parts of an assessment? Can they cope with relatively lengthy instructions? It is obviously crucial to note whether a child has failed a particular item just because the language has been processed ineffectively and therefore the task has not been fully understood or whether they simply could not cope with the information processing involved in the item itself.

Thirdly, distractibility, restlessness and attention deficit disorder per se, with or without hyperactivity, manifest themselves in a significant number of dyslexic children, often with devastating repercussions. In many ways the brighter the children, the more they may be impaired in their functioning. The intellectual elite respond quickly and with considerable insight in problem solving, although they may need to remain on task for several minutes to do so. Attention-deficit individuals, especially the younger children, may well find that attention survives for little more than 30–40 seconds. Their entire level of information processing then deteriorates dramatically. As with their intellectual peers, they may need double this time or even more to reach a solution and yet so seldom have access to this level of concentration. It is almost as though they are unable to access the top 20% of their IQs. Only when they are at a very high level of arousal and thoroughly motivated will glimpses of their brilliance be apparent. The effect on standardized testing is predictable and their ability to cope with classroom work equally impaired (Barkley, 1990; Levine, 1987).

In these instances, I feel that management of the attention deficit is essential for effective further progress and it must therefore be dealt with as a matter of some urgency. My first recommendation would be to look very carefully at diet, as there is increasing evidence that factors in children's food influence their distractibility. I am particularly concerned that they should avoid cola drinks, fruit juices, both apple and orange, dairy products, but only in excess, chocolate products, including sweets, biscuits, spreads, drinks, etc., excess sugars, overflavoured and highly coloured sweets and crisps and, finally, wheat-based breakfast cereals. We have seen the most striking changes with the withdrawal of chocolate products and fresh fruit juice especially. Cola drinks are already recognized in many quarters for their capacity to supercharge a small number of children (Feingold, 1976; Taylor, 1994).

If, after a reasonable span of time, possibly some three months, the effect of dietary control is relatively insignificant, then with a small number of children a paediatric referral is the obvious next step. Dr Sam Tucker will deal with this syndrome in his chapter. I would simply add that the difference in a small minority of children has been inestimable following the prescription of appropriate medication. This has increased the child's arousal level effectively, permitting him to become a normally functioning youngster, able to access those vital IQ points that have been unavailable up to this point. I should stress that at Fairley House the incidence of children on medication is seldom more than 2–3% of the school population. The drug is always prescribed by a Paediatric Consultant and managed by the family doctor. While the children may have to be given a tablet during their day at Fairley House, at no time does the school prescribe drugs or vary the treatment regime without appropriate medical advice.

Reports are prepared each term by the child's teacher and sent to the Paediatric Consultant, who also visits regularly to observe the child in class.

Gross and fine motor coordination will be matters of considerable concern to the perceptual and motor department of the school and fine motor skills are very apparent in psychological assessment, especially on the coding subtest. However, children's drawings and, indeed, the way in which they write out the spelling test give a further insight into the effective use of a writing instrument. Observation from the moment a child is met for assessment and brought to the office, the way in which they move around the room and cope with the stairs, how they return to parents, together with brief catching and kicking exercises, are further insights into gross motor development.

While no attempt is made during an initial assessment to plumb the depths of a child's emotional development, as it is felt unwise to arouse quite unnecessary anxieties which there may not be time to resolve, many children do relax and chat amiably about their school day, their brothers and sisters, their friends and their parents. The stresses and strains of their typical day become only too obvious. Isolating a clear focus of stress gives us the opportunity of helping a child with its management. So often our dyslexic children will be in attention-seeking conflict with their siblings and may even perceive themselves as isolated and distanced from their peers in school. Constant failure and the stress associated with waking up every morning knowing that, once again, there is no possibility of coping must bring with it inevitable anxiety. Indeed, the way in which a child copes during an assessment with the stress involved and with the failure which is inevitable, from time to time, adds further insight.

For some children the stress is further magnified by a tendency to fatigue which may have nothing to do with an attention deficit; it may simply be, especially in the latter part of the day, that their 'batteries run down' and they become more and more tired and despairing.

RISK TAKING

There is one final and extremely important element in both the diagnosis and particularly the management of dyslexic children which we must discuss before moving on to concrete examples. Recent research at Fairley House has shown that for a small number of children, their failure to respond and thrive has nothing to do with the profundity of their symptoms. Some youngsters with a mass of quite typical symptoms have actually made the most encouraging headway while others, whose problems seem so nominal, appear to struggle to make even a month's progress.

The consistent factor in this latter group has proved to be an inability to take risks. They have learned over the months and years that to stay safely within the confines of certainty and to avoid embarking on any task which might make them look foolish or force them to confront, yet again, the anxieties associated with failure, keeps them safe and, albeit artificially, secure.

Risk-taking groups have been established at Fairley House with quite remarkable success. This is an area of remediation which lies within the remit of both home and school. Poor risk takers will find themselves ensnared by their anxieties, even on family summer holidays. If they can be challenged to 'have a go' and rewarded for the attempt as much as the outcome, this will have a positive impact on their attitudes in other contexts.

Case studies

It is helpful now to draw the threads of all that has been discussed together in a practical context through the lives of two particular school children.

Simon

NAME: Simon
ADDRESS:

DATE SEEN: 11.10.94
DATE OF BIRTH: 22.08.84
AGE: 10yrs 1mth
SCHOOL:

TEST RESULTS
Wechsler Intelligence Scale for Children III

Full-scale IQ = 102

Verbal Scale IQ = 103		**Performance Scale IQ = 100**	
Information	13	Picture completion	13
Similarities	13	Coding	5
Arithmetic	8	Picture arrangement	7
Vocabulary	12	Block design	13
Comprehension	7	Object assembly	12
Digit span	6	Symbol search	10

Average = 10   Range 1 to 19

Neale Analysis of Reading Ability (Revised):

Accuracy: 8yrs
Comprehension: 8yrs 5mths
Reading speed: Very anxious and hesitant

Schonell Graded Word Spelling Test:

Spelling age: 7yrs 5mths

Illinois Test of Psycholinguistic Ability

Visual sequential memory – perceptual age: 7yrs 10mths

Tests of laterality

Hand – for writing: RIGHT
Foot: RIGHT
Eye: Telescope: RIGHT
      Aperture: RIGHT

Simon is a 10-year-old boy who has been to a local State primary school, where his work has been deteriorating dramatically in recent terms and his behaviour is becoming more and more difficult. At home, he has been complaining of constant headaches, tummy aches and refusing to go to school if he possibly can. His written work is extremely poor, but he seems to be relatively bright. He seldom manages more than half a page and this is often illegible and poorly spelled. He has a very bright older sister, who wastes no time in condemning his ineptitude and making him feel even more silly than needs to be the case. A baby arrived in the family ten months ago and has left Simon feeling very much the typical 'middle child'. He commented on one occasion that, 'I often feel a bit like the meat in the middle of a sandwich!' He complains that his sister teases him constantly, is allowed all the freedom and has far more pocket money, while the baby is given constant attention by his mother and often father, leaving Simon feeling lonely and isolated. It is quite evident that his petty pilfering from his mother's handbag has a clear attention-seeking significance. Furthermore, a late August birthday inevitably makes him one of the youngest and least mature members of his group.

At over 10 years of age his reading age is barely eight and his spelling, when he concentrates, is at a 7½-year-old level. However, he seldom does maintain his attention, especially when he is processing written language. Maths is hardly any better.

The Headteacher is concerned that secondary transfer will impose an enormous strain on Simon and suggests that he should be made the 'Subject of a Statement of Special Needs' under the Education Acts and recommends a visit to an Educational Psychologist.

Simon proves to be classically dyslexic. The discrepancy between the comprehension and vocabulary subtests is considerable, with a vocabulary scale score of 12 and a comprehension score of only 7. It is quite apparent in talking to Simon that he becomes very muddled in expressing himself.

Examination of his very weak written work means that a scale score of only 5 on the coding subtest comes as hardly any surprise. He shows weaknesses of both auditory and visual short-term memory, with a scale score of 6 on the digit span subtest from the Wechsler reflecting his poor auditory memory and a perceptual age of 7.10 on the Illinois subtest aimed at assessing his visual short-term sequential memory. There is further evidence of his difficulties of language processing on the picture arrangement subtest, where another scale score of 7 appears.

As is quite plain from the subtest breakdown, Simon has considerable areas of compensatory strengths on the remainder of the subtests on which he produces scale scores ranging between 10 and 14. His full-scale IQ proved to be 102.

Once the diagnostic conclusion had been reached, discussion of treatment and further schooling took place with both the Psychologist and the Headteacher, Mrs Thomson. Placement at Fairley House was felt necessary to prepare Simon for secondary transfer, probably at 12+. His programme would need to embrace language therapy on a regular basis as well as specialized remedial provision. It was also acknowledged that on eventual transfer back to mainstream education, Simon would be technically held back a year, allowing him to be one of the older, more mature members of his group, rather than struggling with his late August birthday.

Claire

NAME: Claire
ADDRESS:

DATE SEEN: 28.04.95
DATE OF BIRTH: 30.03.86
AGE: 9yrs
SCHOOL:

TEST RESULTS
Wechsler Intelligence Scale for Children III

Full-scale IQ = 119

Verbal Scale IQ = 133		Performance Scale IQ = 96	
Information	14	Picture completion	15
Similarities	18	Coding	6
Arithmetic	12	Picture arrangement	10
Vocabulary	17	Block design	8
Comprehension	16	Object assembly	9
Digit span	9	Symbol search	9

Average = 10   Range 1 to 19

Neale Analysis of Reading Ability:

Accuracy: 9yrs 2mths
Comprehension: 8yrs 11mths
Reading speed: Relatively fluent, but vulnerable comprehension

Schonell Graded Word Spelling Test:

Spelling age: 8yrs 7mths

Illinois Test of Psycholinguistic Ability

Visual sequential memory – perceptual age: 8yrs 4mths

Tests of laterality

Hand – for writing: RIGHT
Foot: RIGHT
Eye: Telescope: RIGHT
      Aperture: RIGHT

Claire was 9 years of age when she was presented for an assessment, a delightful child with a pleasant, eager personality and a very high level of motivation. Her reading appeared comparatively sound, although as the academic demands in her prep school increased and became more complex and she was required to process information at an increasingly sophisticated, abstract level, Claire began to find life more and more taxing. To the alarm of both her parents and the school it was now beginning to look as though she would not be able to cope with the next academic year and her future was becoming worryingly uncertain.

Claire herself expressed bewilderment that she seemed to have been able to cope comparatively easily in the previous academic year but now everything appeared much more difficult.

Claire has a very real information-processing deficit. However, in her case it is of some considerable subtlety and complexity. She demonstrates a partly dyspraxic picture, with a surprisingly poor performance on the block design, together with a weak picture arrangement and object assembly, a very poor coding scale score of only 6 and difficulties with auditory and visual short-term memory. However, despite these vulnerabilities, her full-scale IQ was 119.

In Claire's case, she was well taught in her preschool years, has extremely supportive parents who have helped her a great deal with her reading particularly, excellent early infant experience and as a result mechanical reading and the early stages of written work and mathematics seem to present no problem.

However, she has now reached 9 years of age and her reading age, which was 8½ a year ago, has only moved up some 6–7 months. Her spelling disintegrates dramatically once she begins to process written language and concentrates on the manipulation of her pen, which she finds increasingly difficult. Most worryingly, although she appears to read at over a 9-year-old level, her ability to organize, process and retain information is nowhere near this standard. She is clearly choosing these books for herself and, indeed, being confronted with a similar standard in class and yet is failing to process the information involved. As a result, her comprehension is poor, she becomes muddled by the content and her responses can seem somewhat inappropriate at times.

As far as her written is concerned, I have already discussed her faulty spelling, to which I would add a considerable struggle to organize and process her written work effectively. Stories become almost impossible to plan and often have no real beginning or end, or she will reach the point of a story in the very last paragraph.

Her dyspraxic problems are very apparent in several of the non-verbal or performance items, especially the block design. Dyspraxia will not only contribute to the disorganization of her work, but will also have a dramatic impact on the organization of Claire as a person. She has already been confronted with home-work and preparation for school exams, neither of which she finds easy. She is constantly criticized for revising insufficiently and yet appears to have tried very hard. Her parents have great difficulty in settling her down to her homework and she never seems to know where to begin. In her exams, she constantly misses the point, overwrites and becomes panicky and confused.

At a personal level, Claire's life is chaotic. She never has the right equipment for school and constantly loses parts of her uniform, for example. Claire must realize that personal organization will be a vital part of her therapy. She simply cannot expect to arrive in class with a thoroughly disorganized mind and hope to cope adequately. She is typical of the youngsters dealt with in detail by Ingrid Linge in her chapter. Claire will need the regular input of an Occupational Therapist for several terms.

It is quite apparent that Claire's problems are, indeed, complex. She does need classical dyslexic therapy on her spelling, her grasp of phonics is still imprecise, reflecting a suspect ear, nose and throat history in her early days, and she appears to abandon the spelling rules in a remarkably cavalier fashion.

However, her greatest problem revolves around the organization and processing of symbolic language. She reads mechanically but derives little information from the experience and finds it extremely difficult to construct her own ideas in written form. These will constitute core targets for her remedial work, without which her chances of success in public examinations at 16 and, even more particularly, at 18 would be significantly compromised.

The two children whom we have discussed in an attempt to give our understanding of dyslexia a structure are very typical, but it must be remembered that the 'great chameleon' that this syndrome represents can come in many guises and each must be analysed with total clarity to ensure that the individual's needs are being met effectively.

References

Barkley, R.A. (1990) *Attention Deficit Hyperactivity Disorder: A handbook for Diagnosis and Treatment*. Guilford Press, New York.

Benton, A.L. (1974) *Revised Visual Retention Test: Clinical and Experimental Applications*, 4th edn, The Psychological Corporation, San Antonio, Texas.

Bradley, L. (1988) Making connections in learning to read and spell. *Applied Cognitive Psychology*, **2**, 3–18.

Feingold, B.F. (1976) Hyperkinesis and learning disabilities linked to the ingestion of artificial food colours and flavours. *Journal of Learning Disabilities*, **9**(9), 551–9.

Frith, U. (1985) Beneath the surface of developmental dyslexia, in *Surface Dyslexia* (eds K. Patterson, M. Coltheart and J. Marshall), Lawrence Erlbaum Associates, London, pp. 301–30.

Levine, M.D. (1987) *Developmental Variation and Learning Disorders*, Educators Publishing Service Inc, Cambridge, Mass.

Miles, T.R. (1993) *Dyslexia: The Pattern of Difficulties*, 2nd edn, Whurr, London.

Neale, M.D. with Christophers, U. and Whetton, C. (1989) *Neale Analysis of Reading Ability – Revised British Edition*. NFER-Nelson, Windsor.

Snowling, M.J., Stackhouse, J. and Rack, J. (1986) Phonological dyslexia and dysgraphia – a developmental analysis. *Cognitive Neuropsychology*, **3**, 309–39.

Tallal, P. (1980) Auditory temporal perception, phonics, and reading disabilities in children. *Brain and Language*, **9**, 182–98.

Tallal, P. (1995) *Integrative Studies of Temporal Integration: Discussion*, Academia Rodinensis Pro Remediations, Malta.

Taylor, E. (1994) *The Hyperactive Child: A Parent's Guide*, Optima, London.

Further reading

Baddeley, A. and Hitch, G. (1974) Working memory, in *The Psychology of Learning and Motivation*, Volume 8 (ed. G. Bower), Academic Press, New York.

Baddeley, A. and Lieberman, K. (1980) Spatial working memory, in *Attention and Performance* (ed. R. Nicherson), Lawrence Erlbaum Associates, New Jersey.

Bryant, E. and Bradley, L. (1985) *Children's Reading Difficulties*, Blackwell, Oxford.

Chasty, H.T. (1990) Meeting the challenges of specific learning difficulties, in *Children's Difficulties in Reading, Spelling and Writing* (eds P.D. Pumfrey and C.D. Elliot), Falmer, London.

Cornwall, K., Hedderly, R. and Pumfrey, P.D. (1983) Specific learning difficulties: the 'specific reading difficulties' versus 'dyslexia' controversy resolved. *Occasional Papers of the Division of Educational & Child Psychology of the British Psychological Society*, **7**(3), 1–121.

Feuerstein, R., Rand, Y. and Hoffman, M.B. (1979) *The Dynamic Assessment of Retarded Performers*, University Park Press, Baltimore.

Gilchrist, M. (1995) Linking the symptoms of attention deficit with hyperactivity disorder with carbohydrate and thiamin intake in children. Degree thesis, University of North London.

Howe, J.A. (1989) Separate skills and general intelligence, the autonomy of human abilities. *British Journal of Educational Psychology*, **59**, 3.

Kaplan, E. (1988) A process approach to neuropsychological assessment, in *Clinical Neuropsychology and Brain Function: Research, Measurement, and Practice* (eds T.J. Boll and B.K. Bryant), American Psychological Association, Washington, DC.

Paraskevopoulos, J.N. and Kirk, S.A. (1969) *The Development and Psychometric Characteristics of the Revised Illinois Test of Psycholinguistic Abilities*, University of Illinois Press, Urbana.

Reisberg, D., Rappaport, I. and O'Shaughnessy, M. (1984) Limits of working memory: the digit span. *Journal of Experimental Psychology: Learning, Memory and Cognition*, **10**(2), 203–21.

Schonell, F.J. and Schonell, F.E. (1952) *Diagnostic and Attainment Testing*, Oliver and Boyd, Edinburgh.

Snowling, M.J., Goulandris N., Bowlby, M. and Howell, P. (1986) Segmentation and speech perception in relation to reading skill: a developmental analysis. *Journal of Experimental Psychology*, **41**, 489–507.

Tizard, J. (1972) *Children with Specific Reading Difficulties*, HMSO, London.

Wechsler, D. (1991) *Manual for the Wechsler Intelligence Scale for Children*, 3rd edn, The Psychological Corporation, San Antonio, Texas. (Published in the UK by NFER-Nelson, Windsor.)

3   *The Speech and Language Therapist*

Jeanne Reilly

Jeanne Reilly begins her chapter by explaining how the work of the Speech and Language Therapist has only become a regular part of dyslexic diagnosis and treatment in recent times. As so much of the dyslexic syndrome revolves around phonological weaknesses and difficulties in processing both spoken and written language, the input of the Speech and Language Therapist is absolutely crucial to effective diagnosis and treatment and, indeed, to a greater understanding of the syndrome as a whole.

P.G.

The Speech and Language Therapist and the dyslexic child

While researchers, psychologists and remedial teachers have for a long time worked with the dyslexic child, it is only relatively recently that Speech and Language Therapists have seen that they have a useful role to play with this population of children. The Speech and Language Therapist is trained to help anyone who has difficulty communicating, though the profession's title does not indicate how broad this training is, encompassing not only spoken and written language but all aspects of communication. The ability to communicate is crucial to the emotional and social well-being of an individual. Anything that interferes with effective communication, whether it be spoken or written, can set up a whole range of consequences or 'barriers'. In order to establish literacy skills, a child must be a good listener, a clear thinker and an organized speaker. The dyslexic child is often a poor listener, a disorganized thinker and struggles to put meaning across when speaking. When looking at underlying reasons for the poor development of these particular skills, researchers have become more and more interested in the development of skills in the under-five-year-old, an age group with which the therapist has much experience. Indeed, Speech and Language Therapists who work with preschool children, helping them to overcome speech and language difficulties, can see that some of these children go on to present with problems in learning other basic skills such as reading once they enter school.

When considering the preschool child, the Speech and Language Therapist might be involved in improving the way a child produces and organizes the speech sounds of language. The dyslexic child of school age can also have problems organizing the sounds of spoken language or written language. The early difficulties have not necessarily disappeared, but rather have manifested themselves in a different form. Typically, the speech sounds that the dyslexic child at Fairley House might use incorrectly, or not at all, are included in the following list, although it is not exhaustive: /f/, /v/, /w/, /r/, /th/, /s/, /ch/ and /sh/. Because the problem of understanding the symbols of the language, called **phonology**, is so deepseated, it is not one that can be easily solved. Rather, in conjunction with the learning of the written symbol, the child can come to understand the use of the spoken symbols and rectify, with help, the speech difficulty.

Some children have genuine difficulty articulating or organizing their mouths and tongues to make the correct speech sounds. Actual muscle weakness is called **dysarthria**, while a problem in planning and co-ordinating movement is called **dyspraxia.** It is now recognized that dyspraxia is one of the aspects of dyslexia which can affect how children learn and dyspraxia affects not only speech but also whole-body motor organization. Before working at Fairley House I was involved with young children with speech dyspraxia. With the right help the speech difficulties could be largely overcome but a number of children were always referred back in the second or third year of schooling because they were failing to master the early skills of literacy. Looking back, there is little doubt that I had been helping a speech problem that was the early manifestation of a specific learning difficulty or dyslexia. Though the children had mastered the spoken code of the language, they were unable to master the written code, which requires the child to learn a set of symbols.

There are some preschool children whose problems in producing intelligible speech are not caused by any difficulty in making the speech sounds; in other words they seem to be neither dysarthric nor dyspraxic, rather they are unable to work out how the sounds of the language are organized to give meaning. When describing this problem in relation to speech difficulties, the therapist would call this a **phonological** difficulty. Researchers in the field, such as Vellutino (1980), Snowling (1980), Bryant and Bradley (1985 and Bradley and Bryant, 1978) and Goswami and Bryant (1990), have often described the problem the dyslexic child has in attaching meaning to the written symbol as difficulty with **phonological awareness**. The word 'phono-logical' describes the problem of attaching meaning to sounds or symbols, an aspect of language or communication that is funda-mentally flawed in many dyslexic children. Dyslexic children can be heard muddling words and phrases and yet do not recognize they are doing so.

Apart from the speech problems described above, the therapist working with preschool children aims to improve the communication of children who may be able to speak clearly, but who struggle to get their meaning across. This could be because they cannot think of the correct word to use. This is a problem for some dyslexic children too. Others fail to understand and use language appropriately in a social setting. The inability to understand the social nuances of the spoken language is rec-ognized as one of the frustrations which some dyslexic children experi-ence and it is appropriate for therapists to help in this area of confusion. Learning the grammar or **syntax** of the spoken language is a struggle for some preschool children and there are a very small number of school-age dyslexics who also need help in this area of spoken language.

The therapist is also trained to understand and remediate the prob-lems of listening and attention, which some children exhibit. In the preschool period these are the pupils who do not settle to any game or activity. In the dyslexic group it can range from the highly distractible child, who cannot concentrate in the classroom, to the child who is lethargic and cannot easily be motivated.

If there is a problem with any aspect of verbal communication as described above, there is bound to be a problem putting thoughts onto paper. Written efforts will be no more coherent than spoken ones. Likewise a child who cannot listen to what the teacher is saying in class will not be able to concentrate to learn reading, writing or any other skill. Some children who enter Fairley House are barely ready to cope with literacy, because their verbal and listening skills are so poorly developed. The therapist can help prepare them for learning.

A study of the case histories of children attending the school during one academic year revealed that some 12% were reported by the parents to have had some difficulty in the development of speech sound production, word organization, sentence structure or sequenc-ing of ideas in the preschool years. These early problems may well have been the first indication that some aspects of learning were faulty. Apart from these children, there are a considerable number attending the school at any one time who have some difficulty expressing them-selves clearly and concisely when speaking. Of course, the vast majority of pupils have problems putting their thoughts onto paper in a coherent way. The Speech and Language Therapist therefore has an important role to play in helping the dyslexic child become an adequate listener and oral communicator, which will prepare him to learn the skills of literacy.

Having accepted that the dyslexic child struggles with language in its different forms, it is helpful to establish why the human being uses language. Written and spoken language is used for the following purposes:

- to understand and express ideas;
- to make and maintain relationships;
- to understand and partake in social interaction;
- to understand and express opinions and emotions;
- to control the behaviour of oneself and others;
- to think creatively and solve problems.

In spoken language the non-verbal aspect is as important as the verbal component. This includes facial expression, tone of voice and accompanying body movement, all of which can prove difficult for some dyslexic children to appreciate and use. In the normal development of language skills a child will have considerable proficiency in all the listed areas by the time they reach seven. As the child develops into adulthood these skills are refined to cope with the many different situations in which he will find himself. A dyslexic child may have a problem in any of these areas and any one function affected will influence how well other aspects of learning develop. The language of the dyslexic can, as a consequence, become distorted and complex to unravel.

LANGUAGE AND LEARNING

Language is crucial to learning. Verbal or spoken language is the most important means a child has of learning and functioning in the world. In time, written language is needed in order to function in a different capacity, since it opens up other possibilities to learn, through books for instance. Language, both verbal and written, is a learned or **cognitive** skill. Other cognitive or learning skills which affect or are affected by language include short-term or working memory and reasoning and problem solving. All these cognitive skills are interdependent and the breakdown of one can adversely affect the development of another. The Educational Psychologist assesses cognitive skills, including some language skills, when carrying out an intelligence test. These language assessments, however, will not have the same depth as those which the Speech and Language Therapist conducts. However, the collaborative and complementary roles which the Psychologist and the Speech and Language Therapist play can benefit the dyslexic child enormously. This is discussed further when describing the assessment procedure.

LANGUAGE AND MEMORY

Without language the human being cannot change information into symbols to store in the mind (the **phonological process**). Without the ability to remember information in the mind, the human being cannot learn from experience. The more a child is able to make sense of what he hears or sees, the better he is able to store information in memory. Even rote learning, which may not initially have much meaning for the child, usually has a rhythm to it or a repetitive pattern that helps when memorizing it. Of course, if the dyslexic child finds it difficult to pick out the rhythm or pattern, this will affect learning too. One of the problems which identifies the dyslexic child is the inability to store information in memory.

WORD-FINDING DIFFICULTY

Some children appear to have problems in their ability to find the correct and precise word to use when speaking and might be described as having a 'word-finding' difficulty. These children can be identified as being difficult to follow in conversation. They use 'he', 'she', or 'them' rather than the name of the person or object. It is very difficult to know whom they are talking about, since they rarely make initial reference to the subject of their story. It may be reasonable to suppose that this problem is also compounded by the inability to store the word in memory in the first instance.

Case study

Jake was a boy of 7 years 8 months and a verbal IQ of 91 who had great difficulty expressing himself adequately in words. When telling a story from pictures or describing his holiday, he used 'he, it and they' so freely that it was almost impossible to follow his description. The listener had to ask questions constantly in order to keep track of what he was describing. While Jake could draw what he wanted to say, he could not label the concepts in his mind with accurate words. One of his remedial needs was to help him find ways of remembering the verbal labels for important people and aspects in his life. Over time the therapist was able to achieve this, using Jake's own pictures as the basis from which to learn the necessary vocabulary before he attempted to tell his story.

SOCIAL USE OF LANGUAGE

Spoken language is a powerful tool in both understanding and manipulating the environment in which we function. Language gives human beings the ability to reason and solve problems. It provides children with a means of understanding people around them, as well as a medium for thinking creatively and expressing novel ideas. Without good use of language the individual can have problems functioning adequately in the modern world. Children with specific learning difficulties frequently fail to understand the more abstract aspects of spoken and written language. They find it difficult to move from the concrete use and understanding of language to its more abstract use where verbal reasoning skills are involved. This is an area of work familiar to the Speech and Language Therapist. A case study illustrates the problems.

Case study

Andrew had a verbal IQ of 138. In spite of this and a very good knowledge of the meaning and use of individual vocabulary, his social use of language was poor. During any group discussion he would take command and monopolize the discussion. As far as he was concerned, once he had the teacher's attention there was no reason to release it. He would simply not notice when other children tried to interrupt. Children in the group were frustrated by this behaviour, but did not know how to handle it. He was genuinely surprised when it was pointed out to him that the aim of the discussion was to give everyone a chance to talk and that one of the duties of the group members was to be aware of when it was time to let others have their say. The Speech and Language Therapist's role here was to teach Andrew how to function as a group member. His high verbal IQ was only an indication of his good understanding of words and ability to reason through problems, not an indication of how he used this language socially.

The role of the Speech and Language Therapist in helping children with these problems is often not immediately recognized. The use of language to make and maintain relationships and to understand how we all relate to one another can be very difficult skills for some children to learn. Not only do they fail to 'read' facial expression and tone of voice, but they may also miss a play on words which is meant as a joke. Colloquial expressions and commonly used phrases can also be lost on these children. This can lead to a great deal of misunderstanding, confusion and unnecessary offence being taken by some children. The use of role play in groups, as well as help in understanding and using the subtleties of social language, are two ways the therapist might help the dyslexic child.

Case study

Another aspect of this kind of help is illustrated by Ed, who was having enormous difficulty keeping his slightly older sister from coming into his room and taking his books and toys. It took some time for the therapist to help this boy explain what was happening and how angry he felt about the situation. The use of dolls and dolls' furniture was found to be the best way of understanding and helping the difficulty. Through role play, using the dolls, Ed could pretend he was in the situation at home with his sister. He could physically control his sister and the 'door' to his room, as well as acting out his part with the therapist (who played the part of the sister) in all the different scenarios. Gradually he learned to transfer what he was playing out in therapy to the real situation at home. With the help of the therapist he was able to put his thoughts and feelings into words and learn to have more control over the situation at home.

LANGUAGE, ATTENTION AND LISTENING

The ability to be attentive and to listen to language is vital in the learning process. In order for an individual to understand the world they need to be able to pick out sounds in the environment and understand what they signify. So for example, a baby learns that a bark is the sound of the family dog or cutlery on the table means it is time to eat. Learning about these sounds takes place at the same time as a child is learning to recognize the sound of voices and to appreciate tone and rhythm in the human voice. Within the first year of life a baby makes the connection between specific words and the meaning attached to them. The words 'good girl', 'clap hands' and 'bye bye' soon have meaning beyond their rhythm. In order for a baby to learn the meaning of words he needs to be able to pick them out from all the other sounds occurring at the same time in a noisy environment. The skill of being able to 'attend' or be ready to listen develops through known stages during the first six or seven years of life. By the time a child reaches school age he should be able to pay attention in class, to listen to the teacher's instructions and then act upon them.

Some dyslexic children, however, do not reach a sufficient level of attention to allow them to cope in class. They never seem 'ready' to take in verbal instructions, having their attention distracted easily. At the other extreme they may become visually or aurally 'fixated' on a particular aspect in their environment. They then cannot be easily aroused to attend to instructions. The effect of either situation is that the child is 'unavailable' for learning. Some dyslexic children have a real and persistent problem with maintaining concentration. The development of listening and attention seems to have stopped at a stage well below their chronological age.

Case study

Antony, at age 8 years (verbal IQ 86), would be transfixed by something happening in the class, quite unable even to respond to the calling of his name. He found it very hard to work out where different sounds in his environment were coming from since he had not learned which ones to respond to and which ones to ignore. It was only when his visual and auditory attention could be harnessed at the same time that he could move from his fixed attention point. Antony, at age 8, had an attention level equivalent to that of a 3-year-old. Helping him to develop age-appropriate listening and attention skills was the priority for the Speech and Language Therapist.

EXPRESSIVE LANGUAGE PROBLEMS

While many dyslexic children are highly articulate and verbally competent, some have great difficulty putting their thoughts into a verbally coherent form. They may not be able to store or retrieve words in their memory for future use. They can be confused when understanding or using the grammar (or syntax) of spoken language. If spoken language is impaired, then it follows that written language will reflect the same problems. In an educational environment, where Speech and Language Therapists are on site, they can and do work closely with the class teacher to improve the spoken language skills of the dyslexic child. Some problems are more appropriately dealt with by seeing the child in an individual lesson, while other needs relating to expressive language problems can be tackled in group lessons. The 'Speaking and Listening' element of the English syllabus of the National Curriculum is covered at Fairley House under the direction of the Speech and Language Therapist.

Case study

Simon, with a verbal IQ of 113 and exhibiting average ability to describe the meaning of words, could not put his thoughts into a grammatically correct spoken sentence. At age 8, and with a verbal IQ of 113, he did not use the verb 'is' correctly in his spoken or written language. He would say 'He sitting next his Mum', missing out the all-important use of 's' at the end of 'he'. Simon could not correctly demonstrate comparative size by using the word ending 'er' so he would say 'He more tall', rather than the grammatically correct 'He's taller'. Simon's early speech and language development had been slow and even at 8 years he was still learning the syntax of his own language. The therapist first had to teach Simon how to 'listen' for particular word endings. Then the work aimed to give Simon practice situations so he could try out the new patterns of spoken sentences.

THE SPEECH AND LANGUAGE THERAPIST AS PART OF A TEAM

The therapist working with the dyslexic child will do so effectively only as part of a multidisciplinary team where each member offers specialist knowledge. The Speech and Language Therapist has long had a working relationship with the Educational Psychologist in the assessment of children and the planning of remedial programmes. More recently in this country, the Occupational Therapist has become part of this team, offering the Speech and Language Therapist further insight into how motor and visual aspects of learning affect speech and language development. The class teacher understands how the child learns in the group setting and how to teach the curriculum in the group situation. The therapist relies on the teacher to evaluate the child's skills in these areas and to make use of the therapist to support the child in individual or group lessons.

The remedial teacher and the Speech and Language Therapist both focus on helping to remediate specific problems so the child can function better in the class and have access to the curriculum. While the Speech and Language Therapist will be especially concerned with skills which support verbal language, the remedial teacher's remit is to support the written language skills. Of course, the dividing line between these two professions is not as clear as that and it is to everyone's benefit that it is not. An overlap might occur when the therapist is developing listening skills in a child, using the written word to back up the work and seeking guidance from the remedial teacher as to appropriate written work to use. On the other hand, the therapist would advise the remedial teacher on realistic ways to gain and maintain a child's attention during a remedial lesson. The parents are also members of this team and can back up the work carried out in school, while seeing their child's progress from another point of view.

The Speech and Language Therapist and the class teacher

Working in the classroom as part of 'team teaching' makes the relationship between the therapist and teacher a close professional one. In the core lessons of maths, reading and phonics or literacy skills, they will both come to know and understand the children very well over the course of an academic year. Both try to adapt their teaching to help the children gain access to the curriculum. The therapist can develop a clear picture of how children function in class and how their therapy can aim to make life and learning in the class easier.

The Speech and Language Therapist's role in assessment

An integral part of a Speech and Language Therapist's work is that of assessment. Before any child is accepted at Fairley House, a multidisciplinary assessment is carried out by the Educational Psychologist, the Occupational Therapist, the Headteacher and the Speech and Language Therapist. The parents play a part in this assessment through the information they provide in the questionnaire. Each team member has a unique understanding of the child and each paints part of the picture of the child's strengths and weaknesses from their own particular professional viewpoint. It is essential that the child is evaluated in different ways because of the complex nature of dyslexia.

The Speech and Language Therapist's conclusions are formed not only from the assessments they carry out, but from the assessments and conclusions of the other team members since there are common areas of assessment and interest between the professionals. So, for example, the Psychologist will, as part of the Wechsler (1991) procedure, investigate verbal reasoning skills. The Speech and Language Therapist also looks at verbal skills but in more detail, with particular reference to the use a child makes of this verbal ability in communication. The Occupational Therapist, in their evaluation of the child's fine and gross motor functioning, can provide the Speech and Language Therapist with information relevant to the speech articulation of the child. The Head, as a teacher, looks at the way the child applies skills to access the curriculum. This information is very important to the Speech and Language Therapist, who needs to judge how communication skills would affect the child in any learning situation in school. The questionnaire the parents provide gives essential information as to the early development of the child, including the early speech and language development.

Once all the members of the team have seen the child, one of the most valuable parts of the assessment process takes place. This is the case conference, when the Educational Psychologist, the Speech and Language Therapist, the Occupational Therapist and the Headteacher meet to discuss and evaluate their findings. From this a decision can be made as to whether the child is suitable for Fairley House. Not every child who attends Fairley House will need to see a Speech and Language Therapist while at the school. They may have been assessed as having good communication skills and would receive help from the remedial teachers rather than the therapist. A typical child who would benefit from the help of the Speech and Language Therapist is illustrated in Fig. 3.1,

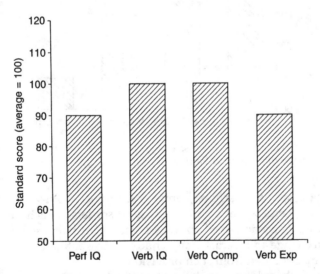

Fig. 3.1 Child A comparative skills. The graph shows the level of verbal skills that would make placement at Fairley House School appropriate.

Child A. This child's verbal IQ (assessed by the Wechsler Intelligence Scale for Children III) and verbal comprehension skills are much better than his ability to express himself verbally. The therapist's aim would be to improve verbal expression so it was at the same level as the other verbal scores.

Children do present for assessment who prove to be unsuitable candidates for the educational environment of Fairley House. These may be the ones who would need a disproportionate amount of the Speech and Language Therapist's time, suggesting that they have a primary verbal communication difficulty. Also daily withdrawal from too many lessons for specialized individual speech and language work could create new problems in terms of missing the curriculum. Often, too, the child who needs this amount of the Speech and Language Therapist's time needs daily sessions from the Occupational Therapist too. Fig. 3.2, Child B, illustrates one for whom alternative school placement would be discussed.

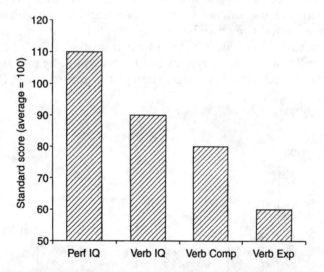

Fig. 3.2 Child B comparative skills. The graph shows the level of verbal skills that would make placement at Fairley House School inappropriate.

There are specialist schools, units and provision for children with significant specific speech and language disorders, which are appropriate for the child described above. Of course, the balance of skills and needs can change and, occasionally, children have entered Fairley House having first benefited from such provision.

Children whose language skills are a little delayed but not severely so can be considered for Fairley House. The criterion for suitability is once again how much language help they would need to catch up and cope in the class. Simon, for example, could not understand and use word endings and shortened words, such as /s/ in 'goes' and 'he's'. He could, by contrast, understand the meaning of words better than most in his class. He had specific difficulties in all areas of literacy, but could cope well with understanding the curriculum subjects.

Should a child's delay in language development reflect a general developmental delay, as measured by intelligence tests, Fairley House would not be a suitable placement.

THE ASSESSMENT

In order to say whether a child would benefit from the school the Speech and Language Therapist needs to look at a number of specific areas of functioning. Both formal and informal assessments have a role to play. The therapist would assess the ability to 'listen and attend' for language, learning, understanding and use of spoken language, and for understanding and use of language in social inter-action, the ability to match the spoken to the written symbol, the ability to remember verbal information in short-term or 'working' memory and speech sound production and use.

The initial speech and language assessment cannot be exhaustive. It is, however, possible to choose the assessments carefully so that a conclusive decision can be made, with the other assessment team members, as to the needs of the child. Some of the children who are accepted into the school will need further indepth assessment which will form part of the basis of the remedial programme for them.

The case conference works well to foster the growth of understanding between all of those involved. After agreement is reached, the feedback of information from the assessment is given via the psychologist and the Headteacher. Any assessment results need to be explained to the parents and should indicate the degree of difficulty the child is experiencing in the areas assessed so that realistic goals can be set. When there are very specific and complex speech or language disorders to be explained the therapist would relay this to the parents direct. The Speech and Language Therapist provides a full written report of the assessment for the parents.

The combined information from all the individual members of the team will provide a clear picture of the strengths and weaknesses of the child and therefore where remediation should begin. These assessments are a 'snapshot' of the child at one particular time. In order to take a fresh 'snapshot' while the child is attending the school, further assessments will be carried out. This is achieved in a number of ways where the therapist is involved. For example, children have a regular annual review, as part of which, the Speech and Language Therapist reassesses children in their areas of weakness, using the original tests for comparison when appropriate. This is a way of judging how therapy and remediation have helped and is a basis for planning further help. Reassessment may take place at other times if there is particular concern regarding an aspect of the child's behaviour or learning. This may be instigated by a member of staff or by the parents. An annual reassessment is also required as part of the legal requirement if children have a 'Statement of Special Educational Needs'. This is provided by Fairley House for the local education authorities and again, the Speech and Language Therapist may be involved as appropriate in this process.

Tests and assessments used

In order to assess the child's difficulties and needs and to plan the programme of remediation, the Speech and Language Therapist can draw on both formal and informal assessments. A formal test will compare a child with others of similar age and will have been tested on a large group of children, while an informal assessment is based on the therapist's knowledge and experience and is a descriptive assessment of performance. Screening tests are quick to administer, but will only confirm a difficulty in an area of functioning. An in-depth assessment will take longer to administer but should pinpoint the nature of a difficulty and help in the planning of remediation. Many of the tests and assessments familiar to the Speech and Language Therapist are appropriate for use with the dyslexic child. When working in a truly multidisciplinary environment, it is vital that the therapist's findings take into account the information provided by the other professionals in the assessment team. The close liaison and understanding between the team members mean that each member understands how interdependent are the different skills of learning.

The completed questionnaire provided by the parents for the initial assessment is a very important part of the assessment process. As more is known about dyslexia and how it manifests, more is understood about the signs in the preschool child which may show part of the dyslexic pattern. Asking for information about these early years provides important clues in confirming the diagnosis. Many dyslexic children have had problems with speech or language development and use before they reach school. A child who did not say his first word until he was three may have had difficulty coping with language at this early age. This would be a contributory factor when looking for a pattern. Some sample questions from the questionnaire, which are relevant to the Speech and Language Therapist, are illustrated below.

- At what age did the child first use words the family understood? (The answer should be somewhere between 6 and 18 months.)
- Was the child's speech clear enough at three years of age for the family to understand and hold a conversation with him? (If it was not clear to the family, there may have been considerable frustration for both the child and the parents.)
- By the time the child started school could he converse easily with other children of the same age and hold his own in conversation? (A child of this age who cannot talk easily with his peers will lose out socially in school and might become withdrawn or aggressive.)

A description of some of the tests used in assessment follows. The list is not exhaustive but rather representative. Different tests assess different aspects of language so a number of tests would be used with any one child. Some tests are chosen because of their suitability with a particular age range, while others are sensitive in testing a particular skill. Therapists have favoured assessments because of their experience interpreting the results. New tests for use by Speech and Language Therapists are published quite frequently. Each has a particular aspect of functioning and a particular population in mind. It is part of the duty of the therapist to assess the relevance and usefulness of new tests.

Clinical Evaluation of Language Fundamentals – Revised (CELF-R) (UK version) (Semel, Wiig and Secord, 1994)
Age range: 5–16 years

The UK version of this test was published in 1994. It is a comprehensive test which assesses both receptive and expressive verbal language skills. More and more Speech and Language Therapists are choosing to use the CELF-R because of the breadth of skills it tests and the wide range it covers. Subtests can be used selectively so specific linguistic areas can be evaluated. From information available prior to the assessment it is possible to decide which parts of the test should be administered. Since it is a picture of the child which is required and since all members of the team add parts of this picture, it is rarely necessary to carry out the whole of the CELF-R at the initial interview. The test is particularly useful when a child with known specific linguistic needs is attending the school. The test comes into its own since it can be used to plan a relevant remedial programme.

The use of the sentence assembly subtest, where the child is presented with written words on a page, can be inappropriate for a dyslexic child because of the reading involved.

The British Picture Vocabulary Scale (BPVS) (Dunn and Dunn, 1982)
Age range: 2 years 11 months–18 years 1 month

This formal test is used to find out how much spoken vocabulary a child understands. A certain amount of verbal reasoning is required. The longer version of the test gives a more accurate result, though the shorter version is useful if time is a constraint. Understanding of nouns, verbs and adjectives is tested by asking the child to pick the correct picture from a choice of four. When used on the population at Fairley House, the score is often almost identical to the verbal IQ score on the WISC III. When the score is very different from the verbal IQ, particularly when the BPVS score is much lower, it can indicate the child has a more subtle language problem than the WISC can assess. When compared to the verbal score on the WISC, the score can there-fore confirm or question the findings.

Case study

Jo, a boy of 7 years, scored an age equivalent of 5 years 11 months–6 years on the BPVS. This gave him a standard score of 88 when the average score would be 100. However, he scored 102 on the verbal IQ scale of the WISC, so showing a discrepancy between the BPVS and the verbal IQ scores. From the case conference dis-cussion it became clear that Jo had difficulty understanding the vocabulary of spoken language. As part of Jo's remedial pro-gramme in the school the Speech and Language Therapist helped him to learn, understand and use vocabulary in its spoken and written forms. Eighteen months after the initial assessment at 8 years 7 months, Jo's standard score on the BPVS was 102, indicat-ing that his understanding of vocabulary was now age appropriate and at the same level as his verbal IQ.

The Renfrew Word-Finding Vocabulary Scale (Renfrew, 1988)
Age range: 3 years 6 months–9 years

This particular naming test is familiar to many Speech and Language Therapists. The child is presented with fifty simply drawn, black and white pictures which the child is asked to name. The results cannot be directly compared to the BPVS which is a test of comprehension of vocabulary, since the Renfrew test uses only nouns. When a dyslexic child cannot name the pictures they might be able to describe them and the indication might be one of the recall of names.

It has been recognized for some time that a naming test for children with a wider age range is needed. There are some American tests which may be worth using to try to fill this gap.

The Renfrew Action Picture Test (Renfrew, 1986)
Age range: 3 years 6 months–8 years 5 months

This is a screening test rather than an in-depth test and was designed to look at how children used sentences in their language. The ten colour pictures the child is asked to talk about appeal to most children. The sentences the child uses to describe the pictures are scored for use of information and grammar in the spoken replies. Listening to a child's language in conversation with the tester is an informal way of assessing a child's skill in sentence construction.

The Test for Reception of Grammar (TROG) (Bishop, 1983)
Age range: 4–11 years

The Test for Reception of Grammar assesses the understanding of twenty of the most commonly used grammatical (syntactical) structures of spoken English. The child picks out one picture from a set of four in response to a sentence spoken by the therapist. It is a useful screening test for children up to the age of eight. Experience shows that beyond this age the results are not sensitive enough to pick up problems in the typical child referred to Fairley House. The sentence structure subtest of the CELF-R similarly tests the understanding of spoken sentences and seems to be more sensitive in the relevant age group.

The Bradley Test of Auditory Organization (1980) (also known as the 'Odd Man Out' Test)
Age range: 5–7 years

This is a test used more and more by psychologists, remedial teachers and others to assess the ability of children to understand rhyme and alliteration in spoken language. Researchers have established a link in the preschool child between ability to understand rhyme and subsequent literacy skills. In Bradley's test the child listens for sounds within words and is asked which word in a set of four is the 'odd one out', in other words, does not follow the rhyming pattern. For example, in the list 'hat, mat, fan, cat', the word 'fan' does not rhyme with the other three. Some dyslexic children of seven and eight do not even score at the 5-year-old level. While not being conclusive, a low score can help to form part of the whole assessment.

SPEECH

About 12% of children attending Fairley House at any one time have a noticeable, but not major, speech difficulty. A number of speech sounds may not be used appropriately by the child or the speech might be slow and laboured or the child may have difficulty producing the correct stress patterns in multisyllabic words. Information from the questionnaire concerning the early development of speech, language and feeding helps the therapist to trace the history of any spoken language problem. The Occupational Therapist's assessment of motor functioning is also helpful to the Speech and Language Therapist, since some speech difficulties are part of a general motor impairment.

Severe speech difficulties, resulting from dyspraxia, dysarthria and phonological difficulties, can be assessed using specific tests available to therapists for more complex difficulties. They are not discussed here.

LISTENING AND ATTENTION

The ability to attend and listen is a sign of a child's ability to screen out distractions to allow him to learn. Listening and attention go hand in hand, since they are two aspects of the same skill. They are assessed through observation of the child not only by the Speech and Language Therapist, but by all those who see the child on the day of assessment. The stages in the development of attention skills are well described in the book *Helping Children's Language Development* by Cooper, Moodley and Reynell (1978). Reference to these stages can be helpful. When a child enters school at five, he should be able to listen to instructions in class, as well as respond to his name when called. Any child unable to shift his attention with ease from one task to another is at a serious learning disadvantage. Some dyslexic children cannot listen and attend at an age-appropriate level. This is one of the reasons they appear to behave in an immature way, because they are stuck at an earlier stage of development.

In a lengthy multidisciplinary assessment some children concentrate for the first hour, but this may gradually deteriorate until the child is very distractible for the last person completing the assessment. Some have poor attention only when asked to do anything they find difficult and some concentrate well until they eat their packed lunch. The change in the concentration of some children following their lunch is so marked that the implications cannot be ignored. The way that some foods affect behaviour is discussed elsewhere in this book.

SOCIAL INTERACTION

Social interaction is assessed by observation of how the child behaves on the day of assessment. If there are doubts about how a child interacts socially or uses language, the child may be asked to come into school to spend the day with their peers. Any child who is likely to have serious difficulties coping socially at the school will hinder his own learning and quite possibly that of others. This is an area of behaviour of great interest to Speech and Language Therapists and some assessments are gradually coming on the market. The Psychological Corporation are introducing new tests all the time and reference can be made to their catalogue for new additions in these areas of interest.

Linguistic Assessment, Remediation and Screening Procedure (LARSP)
(Crystal, Fletcher and Garman, 1989)
Age range: 9 months–5 years

This very detailed assessment has only limited use at Fairley House. It is time consuming to administer and its particular strength lies in assessing the child under 5 years, although aspects of the assessment are useful with the school-age child. It is occasionally used when a detailed, in-depth assessment of a child's use of language structures is needed in order to plan remediation.

Case study
Timmy was a 9-year-old boy whose verbal IQ was 118. He wrote complex stories, using excellent vocabulary. However, he did not know how to engage in conversation with either his classmates or his teachers, responding to questions by always answering in one or two words. An analysis of a conversation between him and the Speech and Language Therapist and of his written work, using the LARSP procedure, showed a boy who could write in complex sentences but who seemed unable to speak in complex sentences in a social context. A term of remediation using role-play situations helped Timmy to understand what was required of him in 'conversation' and gave him the confidence to verbalize the complex language he had only used in the written form.

INFORMAL OBSERVATIONS

Having used formal tests it is helpful for the Speech and Language Therapist to ask the child to produce a piece of written work. This can take the form of drawing a picture and writing a word, sentence or paragraph to describe the picture. The comparison between what the therapist knows about the child's linguistic competence and his written competence can then be made. All too often the gap between a child's spoken language and his written efforts is much larger than would be expected. Noting a child's reaction to written work can be as telling as the actual piece of work he produces.

HEARING

A hearing test may have been carried out on a child before he comes for assessment. The questionnaire asks for details of tests and their out-come. Children who have suffered frequent ear infections may have had several hearing tests. Those who have had 'grommets' inserted in their ears to alleviate middle-ear problems will certainly have been tested. All children new to Fairly House have a pure tone hearing test and a middle-ear function test known as an 'impedance' test. A hearing test assesses a child's ability to hear sounds, but it does not test how a child interprets these sounds in the brain or how well they concentrate. These tests simply show if there is a specific problem in the middle ear or the auditory nerve.

Reynell Developmental Language Scales (Reynell and Huntley, 1993)
Age range: less than 12 months–7 years

This screening test is rarely used at Fairley House. Its strength lies in its use with the under-5-year-old. However, it has proved a valuable tool with children who come for assessment and present with serious delays in verbal comprehension and expression. It can indicate a language age which is below the level of acceptance for Fairley House.

IN-HOUSE TESTING

The Speech and Language Therapist will retest children from time to time, as part of the annual review or to accompany the annual Statement of a child, or to judge whether an intervention procedure has achieved its aims.

The Speech and Language Therapist's role in remediation

The Speech and Language Therapist at Fairley House School enjoys a varied role. This is not only because the therapist works in so many different teaching situations with the children, but also because she works in a truly multidisciplinary environment. The therapist can work with children on a one-to-one basis, as well as in small groups in and out of the classroom. The opportunity can occur for a therapist to see a child in as many as nine or ten lessons per week. Problems which can occur with trying to transfer skills taught in one teaching situation to another can therefore be addressed.

THE THERAPIST AND THE CURRICULUM

Any curriculum subject can form the basis of remedial work and in its turn can support classwork. For example, Charles wrote a weekly diary in his remedial lesson with the Speech and Language Therapist. This followed his craft, design and technology lesson where he was making a kaleidoscope. The aim of the lesson was to develop his poor ability to recount verbally real events in preparation for writing about them. Handwriting, which was being taught by the Occupational Therapist, was also incorporated into the lesson. Over the term Charles came to enjoy what had been a trial at the beginning of the term. He surprised himself in his achievements and he set his own goal of writing a weekend diary the following term, something he would have been quite unable to contemplate initially.

THE THERAPIST AND 'SPEAKING AND LISTENING'

Historically at Fairley House the Speech and Language Therapist has taken charge of addressing the speaking and listening needs of the children. Long before the instigation of the National Curriculum, Fairley House School placed great importance on these skills and saw the need for children with specific learning difficulties to be taught how to listen, attend and develop their ability to express themselves verbally. Since the advent of the National Curriculum, the school has sought to develop its own speaking and listening programme for the dyslexic child.

THE THERAPIST AS CLASSROOM SUPPORT

The therapist at Fairley House often finds it necessary to be in the classroom, working to support the teacher in a maths lesson, for example. The teacher she supports will be the trained maths teacher who determines the content of the lesson, but it may well be the therapist who identifies an individual child who is having problems. In a successful working team both teacher and therapist will see that the partnership can be an equal one. The therapist may identify a child who is having difficulty interpreting questions. Whether the child is having trouble with maths concepts or with the language used in maths problems can be investigated by the teacher and therapist together. A child might have difficulty discriminating between similar sounding numbers, such as 'seventeen' and 'seventy'. The therapist can also help a child to understand some of the vocabulary used in maths, e.g. the different words used to indicate addition, i.e. plus, total, altogether, add, sum of. The combined creativity of two teachers working together to tackle specific learning difficulties in maths is of benefit to the children and allows for fresh insights into how children learn.

Group lessons in phonics and reading at Fairley House are organized so that small groups of children can be taught in two of the key areas of their needs. Depending on previous training and experience, the Speech and Language Therapist may take a group phonics or a group reading lesson. Initially a new therapist will be teamed with an experienced member of staff, before taking a group alone. The Speech and Language Therapist brings to Fairley House a specialist background in specific areas such as specific language difficulties, specific speech disorders and problems with social language and interaction (also known as **pragmatics**). All of these difficulties can and do occur in the dyslexic child and can be tackled in individual and group situations at Fairley House.

LISTENING AND ATTENTION SKILLS

The ability to hear and understand sounds begins with environmental sounds and soon includes the sounds of speech and all its meaning. The skill of attention is that of controlling and focusing the ears and eyes to listen and watch. This skill starts to develop as soon as the child is born and continues through the early school years. Being able to listen and attend at an age-appropriate level is vital if children are to learn to understand the sounds of speech and then the sounds of letters for reading. Since one of the known difficulties of the dyslexic child is the inability to attach meaning to sounds for reading, it is not surprising that the skill of understanding sounds in the environment can also be a problem.

The Speaking and Listening section of English in the National Curriculum (Department for Education, 1995) offers useful suggestions and guidelines for developing these skills in children. Gradually more and more material is being produced to provide resources for therapists and teachers to develop these skills and to help children who have real difficulties in these areas. Some ideas for remediation are given below. In an environment such as Fairley House the emphasis of the work in this area might be different to the stages of the National Curriculum because of the much greater delay in the development of these skills for the dyslexic child.

Ideas for remediation

Work can often be done in groups, since this is the situation where the distractions occur. The element of competition is also helpful in a group, where the skill of learning to listen is interactive. Some children need to learn the fundamental difference between sound and silence. In advanced activities the children can listen to taped instructions which they must carry out. Persuading the child to have control over his behaviour is very much a part of the learning process.

There are commercially produced books and activities which provide excellent resources for lessons. Many of the activities are used in nursery schools. Musical statues and 'Simon Says' are two such examples. These can be adapted for the dyslexic child in school by using musical instruments and letting each child take turns to control the game. 'Simon Says' can be adapted for children listening to common classroom noises. The American Evan-Moor books, published in Britain by Scholastic, include amongst other material a helpful book of ideas called *Listening Skills*, in which is contained not only games to develop listening skills but also pictures for the teacher to use in listening activities. LDA produce a number of taped programmes to improve listening and comprehension, while Schofield and Sims produce the *Oracy* taped listening programme, with the National Curriculum in mind. Taskmaster also publish some useful material.

Group listening and attention programme weekly lesson

A sample programme of help is outlined. It worked with one particular class of 7- and 8-year-old children at the school whose attention levels ranged from a typical 4-year-old to a typical 7-year-old. The half-hour lesson took place once a week over a period of a term and a half.

Sounds in the environment. Begin by asking the children to be silent for a very short time, such as 15 seconds. During this time ask them to listen for a particular sound in the environment such as a car driving past or someone walking along the corridor. Suggest the sounds and name them so there is no confusion, then ask the children to offer their suggestions. Choose familiar classroom sounds to begin, then introduce a less familiar sound such as a box of staples being dropped on the desk.

Listening and talking. This is more difficult because the child is carrying out two skills at once. Decide on a sound to listen for. Engage the class in an activity. When the children hear the sound they should all stop and look at the therapist. Offering to give an appropriate reward will help the children to control their behaviour.

Making sounds. With eyes closed, the children listen for sounds the therapist makes, such as turning the pages in a book, and then try to identify them. The children could try to describe the sound.

Locating sounds. Finding the source of a sound is easier when there are quiet surroundings. Locating them in a noisy classroom is much more difficult. Firstly show the children what sound they are to listen for. With their eyes closed and in silence they listen for the sound and point to where in the room it is being made. In the everyday classroom the child is constantly trying to pick out relevant sounds.

Guessing sounds. This requires more general knowledge about sounds. Into a metal or plastic box, put an everyday object. A paper clip or a staple are examples. Give rewards for having a guess, not just for guessing correctly.

Holding still. The idea is that everyone in the class sits still and silent with eyes closed for a specified amount of time which can increase as the children get better at 'holding still'. If the children hear any neighbour make specific noises such as a cough, shuffling their feet, rocking on their chair, etc., they can point to the neighbour who is then 'out'. Breathing noises are allowed. In this game the children become more aware of themselves and others as makers of sounds. They are beginning to control their own bodies, a difficult task for the easily distracted child.

Understanding rhyme. Much of the recent research has shown that one of the fundamental skills needed by children in order to appreciate the written word is to understand rhyme in the spoken word (Bryant and Bradley, 1985). Young nursery-age children show their understanding in the nursery rhymes they learn. Recognition of rhyming sounds is often a particular difficulty for the dyslexic child.

Teach children to understand the concept of listening for rhyming words. This can be done individually or in groups. Supporting the listening work by showing the written patterns is useful. The patterns do not have to be within the spelling ability of the children. A group of children still working on Consonant Vowel Consonant combinations in their spelling lessons came to appreciate the rhyme 'old' with the help of the pattern being written on the white board. The group was able to add sounds and letters to the beginning of this pattern to produce bold, cold, fold, gold, hold, sold, told. There is now evidence from a number of researchers, including Goswami and Bryant (1990), that normal children understand about these letter patterns before they understand about individual letters and sounds. The research shows that this skill of understanding 'chunks' of words can be taught. At Fairley House initial trials with this approach have been encouraging. Using rhyming poems with a regular rhythm and a predictable word is another way of helping children to understand in the first stages. Written exercises where words are left out, called 'Cloze procedure' exercises, using poems are helpful for children with sufficient knowledge of the written word. Card games with rhyming word endings are commercially available or can be made by the children.

Much more importance is now being placed on the value of young children learning and being taught to appreciate rhyme and rhythm in the language, which is part of how children appreciate the phonology or meaning of speech. Gradually more formal resources for these activities are being produced, which use many traditional ideas and approaches. Nevertheless, there is value in being specific in the help that is given when the process of learning these skills is faulty.

ORAL LANGUAGE SKILLS

Thoughts must be formed in the mind before they are spoken. These thoughts need to be clearly organized if they are to be communicated verbally to others. This can only happen if the thoughts can be transferred into words. This process usually develops without difficulty as the child learns his own language but in the dyslexic child this can present a problem. The consequence is poor ability to organize words and ideas in the mind, with verbal expression being disorganized too. It is insufficient to work on the poorly organized writing skills of dyslexic children when the organization of thoughts and spoken language is the root cause of the problem. Paradoxically, while many dyslexic children are excellent talkers, they are not always good communicators.

The Speech and Language Therapist's skills in understanding spoken language, its development and how it can go wrong are invaluable when working with the dyslexic child. The oral language skills programme at Fairley House School is supervised by the Speech and Language Therapist. The lessons are normally group lessons, although it has proved helpful with some children to use an individual remedial lesson to develop oral language skills if the child has particular difficulty. The aim of the oral language skills programme is to take the child from the first stages of organizing thoughts to follow a simple sequence of events to the stage of using different ways of talking for different situations. For example, the language used in advertisements, in interviews and in debating an argument will all be different in style.

The terms 'speaking', 'talking', 'oral language' and 'verbal expression' all describe the act of putting thoughts into words to communicate to others. The other side of this is 'listening and attention', which must develop first. The remedial aims in this area are as follows:

- to teach the child what is expected of a good communicator;
- to teach the child to organize his thoughts for speaking;

- to teach the child to be a clear verbal communicator;
- to help the child understand his own particular strengths and weaknesses in talking;
- to teach children to work with one another to this end;
- to develop the child's oral language skills to a level where he can transfer this to written language.

The use of tape recorders and video equipment in oral language skills lessons has proved enormously beneficial. Learning to operate tape recorders is in itself a skill of organization and it takes time for children to learn how to do so independently. The tape recorder allows the children to tape their own stories or descriptions and to listen to their efforts. They can then judge for themselves whether they have made themselves clear. With each exercise, aims are set and these are the criteria by which the child judges his recording. So, for example, in a picture description exercise the group might decide on six aspects which must be included in the description. These would be written down as a checklist for the child to refer to while recording. On listening to the tape, either the child or a partner would listen and tick off the items on the checklist. There is generally no writing required in this lesson. It is initially far too complex to organize the verbal language, operate the tape recorders and write notes. Notes can be written by the teacher to draw together discussion. They can then be photocopied so each child can refer to them while recording.

Activities

Examples are given of activities which have been used for children aged 7–12 years in the oral language skills lessons.

Seven-year-old group. Based on a story in picture form, a group of children makes up a story for recording. Each child says one or two sentences only for his picture. Attention must be paid to what has already been said in the story to keep it consistent and this is an important listening component in this exercise.

Nine-year-old group. The children are given five words on a piece of paper around which to create a story. The words have to be introduced into the story in the order in which they are written on the paper.

Eleven-year-old group. Children work in groups of two or three to produce an advertisement for video or tape recording. The group must work together to plan and execute the advertisement. The advert must be presented to the other members of the class for their comments as to how well it would sell the product being advertised.

Twelve-year-old group. Set up interviewing situations to help the children prepare and practise for school interviews.

Curriculum-related activities

In collaboration with the class teacher, the oral language lessons can support curriculum work. These examples have all been tried out successfully.

1. Record the sequence of events in the most recent science experiment. Draw pictures as a plan prior to recording.
2. In conjunction with the design and technology teacher, prepare the children for the week's lesson by discussing the equipment and materials to be used. Then record an explanation of the lesson for another group to judge for clarity and accuracy.
3. Encourage each child to record a piece of his own creative work for other children in another class to listen to.
4. Choose a picture story book which would interest the youngest pupils in the school. Ask an older group to read or tell the story from the pictures, then give it to the younger pupils to listen to as a taped story.

The focus of the oral language lessons can take account of individual difficulties a child is experiencing. A child with specific difficulty putting thoughts into words can be supported by giving him more help to learn the vocabulary of specific subjects. Organizing and memorizing of such vocabulary is the first step towards being able to use it in spoken language. The class teacher and oral language skills teacher can help one another with ideas.

Another benefit of the oral language skills lesson is to foster the ability of those children who are adequately organized in their thoughts and spoken language but whose literacy skills are a long way behind. The lesson can provide them with a vehicle to tell stories, give descriptions, etc. at a level which they would not be able to achieve on paper. For these children a scribe might be used to write down a description or story related on tape, so giving them written credit for their expressive ability.

THE FIRST STAGES OF READING AND SPELLING

Once a child can understand sounds in the environment he can be taught to sort sounds in words. Two skills are involved: firstly, that spoken words are understood to have sounds within them and secondly, that these spoken parts can be represented by symbols. In effect two codes are involved, the spoken and the written code. For the dyslexic child learning either of these codes can be a tremendous struggle.

Since the letters on the page give no clue as to what they represent, this has to be learned. Teaching the letter sounds is a first step. Indeed, children do not have to know all of the sounds of the alphabet in order to make words. Nor do they need to know the letter names as well as the sounds to begin the process. Lyn Wendon, in her Letterland programme (published by Letterland), suggests learning a mere 14 sounds initially. The Speech and Language Therapists at Fairley House have devised and developed a useful means of bridging the gap between the spoken and written symbols of the language. It involves a caterpillar hungry for letters, sounds and words.

The caterpillar

This idea appeals to children up to about the age of eight. The caterpillar has a succession of stomachs or tummies in which he can store either letters or letter combinations. These letters are in the correct order to make words. Some tummies can take only vowels and some only consonants. Putting the wrong vowel into the vowel tummy gives him indigestion and the only remedy is to feed him the correct vowel. Putting a consonant where a vowel should be makes him sick. The caterpillar can be used initially to place a sound at the beginning or the end of a word in a listening exercise. He can be used to spell words where the therapist draws the correct caterpillar length indicating which tummy needs a vowel. He can be used to read words by feeding him a word the child finds difficult. Sometimes a child can read a word using the caterpillar when he cannot break the word down from the text. The caterpillar is extremely helpful in showing visually the direction of letters in words. Words such as 'beginning, front, start, head, first' are used to describe the initial letter position. He can show the shortest of words such as 'in' and progress through Consonant Vowel Consonant combinations such as 'tap' can be illustrated (Fig. 3.3).

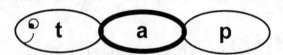

Fig. 3.3 Consonant Vowel Consonant combination.

To overcome the problem of the caterpillar becoming too long, letter combinations, e.g. 'sh', and word endings, e.g. 'ing', can be put in a single tummy, as in the example word 'shopping' in Fig. 3.4. He can be used to show syllables too, as in 'in + side' (Fig. 3.5).

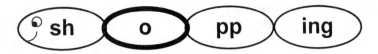

Fig. 3.4 Letter combinations and word endings.

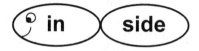

Fig. 3.5 Syllables.

Once a child finds the caterpillar model useful, he will make suggestions as to how to use it. When he finds it quicker to work out a word in
his head, the caterpillar usually becomes redundant.

FROM THE SPOKEN TO THE WRITTEN WORD

Progressing from spoken to written language takes time and some effort
for most children. For those with no specific difficulties motivation to
succeed and a gradual grasp of the symbols used to put words down
onto paper keeps them engaged. For the child with a specific difficulty,
while the motivation may exist at the beginning, without that grasp of
the written code failure leads to loss of confidence and eventually avoidance of the activity. Even with children who have begun to understand
the fundamentals of the written word the step from a concept to its
expression on paper can be so laborious that there is little reward at the
end. In the time it has taken some children to write down a single simple
sentence they have forgotten the train of their thought and have written
something which does not make much sense to either themselves or the
reader.

At this early stage of writing, some children are trying to combine so
many newly learned skills – thinking of ideas, transferring them into
words, spelling, handwriting and checking – that they simply cannot
succeed in any of these areas. There are ways to help overcome this difficult stage, however, and the use of a specialized tape recorder called
the Language Master (available from Drake Educational Associates) or
other recording devices can ease the load. The Language Master is a
commercially produced specialist tape recorder using a 6-second strip of
recording tape which can be played back as many times as required,

using a repeat button, once a recording is made. This helps overcome the problem of trying to play back a very short recorded piece on a conventional tape recorder. The Language Master can tape one single spoken sentence at a time. The child records a sentence, paying attention to clarity and content. He writes the sentence down, playing it back as often as necessary by using the repeat button, concentrating now on the words for spelling and on handwriting. It can be played back yet again while the child checks what he has written with what he intended to write. This method of working allows the child to concentrate on a limited number of skills at a time. A useful checklist developed by the therapist and a number of children is:

- think about the idea;
- speak the sentence;
- record the sentence;
- play it back as often as is needed while writing the sentence;
- check the completed sentence for words, punctuation, spelling, etc.

The child who finds it difficult to concentrate when writing creatively or doing topic work can sometimes be prepared for classwork using the Language Master during a remedial lesson. One such child, Edwin, who was 7½ years old and had a verbal IQ of 128, exhibited both good verbal skills and an adequate grasp of spelling rules, suggesting he could make an attempt at writing. However he could not 'get down' to written work in the classroom. The Language Master was used to create and write down all the sentences in two particular pieces of creative work. He gained confidence because of his success and found he could produce similar work in the class, without having the Language Master with him, but having the checklist on his desk to refer to.

VOCABULARY – UNDERSTANDING, MEMORY AND USE

Vocabulary means words an individual understands and uses, which are either spoken or written. Before a child learns to read, he will hear and remember words by their sounds, because of their meaning and through using them when speaking. Each time a child hears a word, he learns from the context in which it is used. For example, a word such as 'slimy' has a concrete meaning to do with touch. This meaning has to be well understood for a child to appreciate its more abstract meaning when used to describe a person's character. For some dyslexic children they do not progress beyond the concrete to the abstract. This is why jokes are lost on so many of them and why they misinterpret what is said to them.

The following example illustrates an 8-year-old girl trying to describe a picture of a little girl buying ice creams for all the family and handing over the money to the ice cream man. The child does not use specific words for the people, so making it difficult to follow who is in the picture. She is only able to refer to them as 'he, she, him, her, them'.

> She went to buy the ice creams and she gave it to him. He gave her lots, because she had to take them home for them.

Once a child can read, the opportunity for learning new vocabulary, phrases and ways of expressing ideas opens up. Reading influences the words which are used when talking and vice versa. Reading new words is an incentive to increase knowledge. The ability to work out new words in turn improves reading ability. If the reading process is difficult for dyslexic children, the opportunity to increase understanding and use of vocabulary is reduced.

Yet another way that children learn and remember vocabulary for verbal use is in the act of writing the word, using it in their own creative work. This act of writing words, feeling the physical movement and seeing the pattern of letters, helps the child remember them. So often, though, all these skills which help memory are a struggle for the child with specific learning difficulties.

The involvement of the Speech and Language Therapist can be particularly pertinent when dealing with children who cannot remember vocabulary, because of the therapist's particular training in linguistics and language development. The teacher, remedial teacher and therapist, with their different range of experience, can work out the best approach to remediation, whether in class or in individual sessions.

In a school like Fairley House, the class teacher's approach to introducing new vocabulary will help children who have difficulty in this area. Time is spent discussing new words, demonstrating them by practical means and by accompanying such words with pictures whenever possible. Frequent repetition and reinforcement of new vocabulary occurs throughout the school. There are children for whom even this approach is not enough. These children may have a standard score of well below 90 on the British Picture Vocabulary Scale. If their knowledge is poor, their verbal use will be poor too. It is particularly important to ensure that realistic expectations are made for these children.

Sometimes it is appropriate for the therapist to carry out the work on improving the understanding and use of vocabulary or in directing the remedial and class teachers as to how the class teaching can be adapted. Approaches can be either 'child-centred' or 'curriculum-centred'. The child-centred approach works particularly well in the child under 8 years of age with limited reading ability. A curriculum-centred approach draws on the curriculum subject words that the child needs.

Some child-centred suggestions are given below:

- The child, parents and remedial teacher develop a scrap book to include all the things that are important to the child at home and at school, including friends, pets, hobbies, likes and dislikes.
- Undertake a holiday project on a particular subject.
- Keep a log of words the child wants to know more about. This might show a pattern to the problem words.
- Make up quiz questions for the family based around the vocabulary being learned.
- Draw a set of pictures around some of the words and then tell the story on tape to be listened to by the child and their peers.
- Keep a log book of words that cause difficulties, drawn from the reading book, for example. For one child this showed that there was a pattern of words which were not understood. For this child dividing the words up into word classes such as 'doing words', 'naming words', 'describing words', was the key to her being able to file new words in her memory.

Any approach should aim to make the child take some responsibility for learning. Pictures should be used as 'aides-mémoire', so that whoever is talking to the child has a common point of reference and does not feel at a loss.

In a curriculum-based approach the most pressing need may be for the child to understand and keep up with the vocabulary of the different subjects. When introducing this work, either part of a subject area such as science or a topic area such as the Romans could be chosen. Before the term's work begins, the class teacher could give a list of the 'key words' that must be understood and used by the child. Alternatively the class books relating to the subject matter could be made available to the therapist for use in the remedial lesson. In this way the child has a chance of keeping ahead of the new vocabulary rather than always struggling to keep up, which adds to already dented confidence.

Some curriculum-based ideas are suggested below.

- Make a personal picture dictionary for the subject, e.g. science, divided into apparatus, chemical compounds, etc. Alternatively, buy a pictorial science dictionary.
- With the child, make a box file of cards containing definitions of words and add to it as appropriate.
- Draw pictures of word classes, as in a thesaurus, containing not only the new words but also words with a similar meaning, e.g. 'round, circle, sphere, spherical, ball, globe'. Use opposites and similar-sounding words, e.g. 'crumble' and 'crumbly'.
- Learn new words from the root word and add suffixes and prefixes to show how these subtly change words in context, e.g. 'crumb, crumbs, crumbly, crumbling'.

- Present the child with 'Cloze' procedure exercises which the child makes up and gives to another member of the class to try out.

Written work

Using words in written exercises is vital for remembering, understanding and recalling words. For a non-literate child this 'writing' can take the form of pictures. Once the child has begun to understand about letter sounds and names, these can be used to accompany pictures, so forming the link between sounds, a visual image drawn by the child and meaning. Children who are more literate can use their own writing skills to accompany pictures or 'webs' of connecting words as a way of helping with meaning and therefore memory. Where the work of the Speech and Language Therapist ends and that of the remedial teacher begins is hard to decide. The crossover between the two professions should allow for better understanding of the disciplines and of the child. The therapist and the remedial teacher should decide whose time and skills would be best used to help with the transfer of the verbal to the written word.

At the early stages of helping the child with the vocabulary problems described, progress can be slow. Once the best ways of learning and remembering have been identified for the individual child, then progress usually accelerates. Individual learning styles have to be taken into account, if the task is to pay off. Success brings further motivation to learn.

THE GRAMMAR OR SYNTAX OF SPOKEN LANGUAGE

In the same way that some children fail to learn the vocabulary of their spoken or written language, others fail to learn the structure of language, which is called syntax when referring to spoken language and grammar when referring to written language. An example of this kind of problem is illustrated by the child who would say 'He like it' or 'Where the boy gone?' long after he would normally have learned the different uses that 's' has at the ends of words. For other children their difficulty will be in understanding the whole meaning of sentences. They might not understand the sentence 'The boy would have gone swimming with them if he had finished his lunch in time' not because they did not understand the individual words but because they could not piece together all the different dependent parts. While this is not a frequently occurring problem for children at Fairley House, when it does occur its effects can be wide ranging. The understanding of spoken instructions, of text and of social interaction can all suffer. Speech and Language Therapists will be used to seeing these children in 'language units' and in schools for speech and language disordered children. The problem described is not one of the different ways people use syntax in different dialects.

Difficulty in understanding spoken language can leave a child confused in the classroom. When given instructions or when asked questions, the child may respond inappropriately or carry out only part of the instruction or even none of it. These children may not show they have a difficulty in understanding language because they speak in perfectly correct sentences but the sentences they use in conversation, on closer inspection, may not be as complex as one would expect for a child of that age.

Inability to understand the nature of a spoken question or instruction will result in inability to understand written questions and instructions. Understanding text books, written maths instructions and examination questions relies on the child having an ability to cope with the grammar of the questions. If not helped in the spoken form, the written form is likely to remain an area of poor understanding also.

It may be difficult to pinpoint exactly where the difficulty lies when the syntax of spoken language is involved. One reasonable suggestion is that it is, once again, caused by a faulty phonological system, which renders it difficult to attach precise meaning to the sounds of the language. Instead of individual sounds not being understood, it can be combinations of sounds which, when added to words, change meaning, as in: 'retake, jumped, singing, it's, simply'.

Where word order causes children difficulty, it may be that memory is overloaded. The child might not be able to hold the information in short-term or 'working' memory long enough to work out the sense of the whole. The sentence 'it would have been too hot to have travelled by bus that day' illustrates several interdependent ideas concerning the weather, the bus and a particular day.

Written work can illustrate the difficulties a child is experiencing. Obtaining a sample of free writing from the child's class can indicate some of the difficulties the child is likely to be experiencing in spoken language. Using the written word to support work on improving syntax is an advantage. Written sentences containing examples being learned can be read and taped by the child. He can then listen to and use the examples as self-dictation exercises. Working on the spoken and written instructions of the school curriculum is important as it makes them immediately relevant. Opportunities for the child to ask and give instruction can also be included. It can easily be seen how this work on syntax crosses into work on social skills, vocabulary, spelling, reading and listening. Difficulties in one area of learning can and often do have an effect on other areas of learning. A multisensory and multidisciplinary approach to helping the problems is all-important.

SOCIAL USE OF VERBAL LANGUAGE

Verbal language is used to make relationships, to understand how others feel and think, to influence those around us and to make sense of the social rules of society. Children learn how to manipulate their environment with language as soon as they start to speak. Even before that, they have begun to learn how facial expression and body gestures are used to express meaning. The importance of this should not be underestimated. By the time a child is five and in school he has developed a sophisticated communication system. This system continues to develop throughout the child's life and into adulthood. Being able to understand the system allows the child and adult to function in the world of people around them, school, home and work. The inability to understand has serious consequences for how the child or adult will be able to take a useful part in these situations.

For some dyslexic children learning the subtleties of verbal and non-verbal language is very difficult. A child who cannot move from the concrete understanding of words and phrases to their abstract meaning will miss the real import of what people are trying to say. Facial expression, tone of voice, hand gesture and body movement all add to this understanding. The consequences for the dyslexic child go beyond his poor understanding of the social situation.

The ways in which the dyslexic child shows poor understanding of social language are illustrated by the following examples.

- He can misunderstand playground phrases which aim to include rather than exclude children from their peers, e.g. nicknames for group members such as 'shorty' or 'slow coach'.
- He can fail to read facial expression and tone of voice for either praise or reprimand.
- He can fail to understand what is implied in phrases such as 'can you help me please?' which is a command, not a question.
- He may have poor ability to take part in conversation or group discussion, being unaware of how to take turns and be a listener as well as a speaker.

Of course, all of these examples can be seen at times in most children as they learn social language. These difficulties, however, persist in the dyslexic child. Some find it very hard to understand all the implied nuances of language. Trying to reason through problems with these children using verbal language can be most trying. It is as if the two parties were talking a different language, which in one sense they are. Speech and Language Therapy is only one of the disciplines involved in helping the child at Fairley House who has poor understanding and use of social language. Collaboration between the Speech and Language Therapist and the Occupational Therapist has led to the setting up of a remediation programme to help these children. Each therapist has a training and background which equip them to look at aspects of development which affect how children behave socially. How this group tackles the problem is discussed more fully in the Occupational Therapist's chapter. There are some children who have needed both the help of the social skills group and individual help from the Speech and Language Therapist to instigate change in their understanding and behaviour. In providing help to an individual child circumstances can sometimes indicate a starting point as the following example serves to illustrate.

Case study

Greg, with a verbal IQ of 93, was 11 years old when he came to Fairley House. His specific learning difficulties included the areas of verbal and non-verbal language. He did not engage in eye contact appropriately with either his peers or with adults. He did not understand what was required in conversation, being monosyllabic in reply to questions. Although he wanted to have friends, he did not know why he had so few and had failed to appreciate that engaging in conversation with his peers would help in this process. In spite of this, he had an image of himself as an interesting and interested person. Greg was included in a group run by the Speech and Language Therapist and Occupational Therapist to help children develop specific social skills. This group helped him to address some of the problems he was having with his peers and to prepare him better for the interviews for his next school.

In the individual remedial lesson the Speech and Language Therapist and Greg practised interviews in a 'role-play' situation. Greg would be 'interviewed' by a variety of different 'Headteachers' and then would become the Headteacher himself. What he found surprising was the need to be able to form an opinion or give a reply in answer to questions he had not been expecting. Greg would wait a long time after the question was asked thinking of a reply, making the person engaged in conversation with him feel uncomfortable. It was the effect of his lack of immediate responses or inappropriate replies which Greg had failed to recognize. Initially difficult to motivate, after a term Greg could handle an 'interview' with smiles and a confidence which helped him to gain a place in the school of his choice. He learned to formulate ideas and express them pertinently. He gained insight, too, into the broader implication of some lines of questioning. The next stage of help was to make Greg feel more comfortable conversing with staff he did not know well and with the younger children with whom he had little empathy. By this stage Greg had the improved insight and motivation to achieve the success he wanted.

Problem solving is the ability to understand a situation and to think beyond the immediate to find a solution. Situations where verbal language is used to resolve a social problem occur daily for any child. There are situations which occur where arguments have to be resolved, such as jealousy amongst friends. Dyslexic children can have the greatest difficulty with these. Teaching children to understand and use intonation patterns, facial expression and body language is vital if they are to save themselves from endless daily difficulty and confrontation. The Speech and Language Therapist, class teacher, drama teacher and everyone coming into contact with these children have a part to play in helping them. Change can be effected over time. A fundamental change in behaviour and a modified view of the world must be achieved and because this is so fundamental, expectations must be realistic. Some children will continue to need help well into their teens.

SPEECH DIFFICULTIES

The roots of speech difficulties in the dyslexic child may lie in dysarthria, dyspraxia or phonological awareness, as described in the first section of this chapter. Somewhere along the way the child's ability to perceive and understand the sounds of the language has failed to develop adequately. Consequently the child's use of speech sounds is impaired. This can be in spite of the ability to articulate the speech sounds when not contained in words. Some dyslexic children are known to have had problems in developing their speech sounds. The speech problems of dyslexics can persist well beyond the age when most children would have mastered all the speech sounds and speech sound combinations of the English language, i.e. about 7 years of age.

Equipping the child with speech patterns which will be acceptable to the members of his peer group and to himself is a primary aim of this work at Fairley House. Work on correct speech production is well worth emphasizing, since if speech patterns are misunderstood, this will affect both reading and spelling skills. Helping speech can help the child to clarify some aspects of reading. This area of remediation is probably the one most easily understood as being the domain of the Speech and Language Therapist. A knowledge of how speech sounds develop and how to help when they develop incorrectly is vital. The work can be done in a group or with individuals or both. Supporting the speech work with written work is of fundamental importance.

Common speech difficulties that dyslexic children experience are described below, although this list is not exhaustive.

- /f/ and /v/ These are both made using the lips and teeth. The subtle difference between the two sounds is not always easy to hear.
- /w/ and /r/ These two sounds cause many children difficulty. Hearing a difference between them is difficult because of the similar way they are formulated. This is a common enough difficulty in young children who are not dyslexic; however, they usually grow out of the problem, whereas some dyslexics do not.
- /ch/ and /sh/ can be hard for some children to discriminate. The similarity in the spelling is an added complication, e.g. march/marsh.
- /e/ and /i/ (short vowels) are similar in their sound and tongue position and some children have considerable problems with them, e.g. peg/pig.

There are a number of aims the Speech and Language Therapist will endeavour to achieve in helping a child overcome a speech difficulty. These are listed below to help understand the reasoning behind some aspects of a Speech and Language Therapist's work.

- To help the child to hear the difference between two similar sounds.
- To teach the letter representation of the sounds.
- To teach that depending on which sound is used, the meaning of the word can change, e.g. chin/shin.
- To teach the child how the sounds are made. It is useful to focus on articulation even when a child has no difficulty in making the sounds. This is because any sensory feedback will allow the child another way of remembering and understanding the sound. This helps to reinforce and is part of a multisensory approach to teaching.
- To introduce words whose only difference is in the sounds being taught, e.g. fin/thin, fat/that.
- To use a stopwatch to increase the speed with which the child can say pairs of words, e.g. how many pairs in 10 seconds.
- To make up phrases, sentences, poems, stories, games, etc. containing these words, all for the child to say.
- To encourage children with speech difficulties to help each other in listening for clarity, accuracy and speed.

- To connect speech to literacy as soon as possible. Occasionally, if a child is not yet secure with the written symbols of the language, it can be advisable not to work on his speech until he has good understanding of the letters of the alphabet.
- To be patient. It will take longer to sort out these speech problems than most expect.

Teachers and parents can support the child with speech sound difficulties. Just because a child can say the speech sounds correctly in therapy does not mean he can use them correctly in conversation. Dealing with speech difficulties needs a sensitive approach, so that the child is not made to feel that he will be corrected each time he tries to talk. Repetition of new patterns practised over time will usually mean that speech difficulties can be improved or resolved, so helping yet another important aspect of verbal communication.

References

Bishop, C.V.M. (1983) *Test for Reception of Grammar*, Manchester.

Bradley, L. and Bryant, P.E. (1978) Difficulties in auditory organisation as a possible cause of reading backwardness. *Nature*, **271**, 746–7.

Bryant, P.E. and Bradley, L. (1985) *Children's Reading Problems: Psychology and Education*, Basil Blackwell, Oxford.

Cooper, J., Moodley, M. and Reynell, J. (1978) *Helping Language Development*, Edward Arnold, London.

Crystal, D., Fletcher, P. and Garman, M. (1989) LARSP procedure. *The Grammatical Analysis of Language Ability*, Whurr, London.

Department for Education (1995) *English in the National Curriculum*, HMSO, London.

Dunn, L.M. and Dunn, L.M. (1982) *British Picture Vocabulary Scale*, NFER-Nelson, Windsor.

Goswami, U. and Bryant, P.E. (1990) *Phonological Skills and Learning to Read*, Lawrence Erlbaum, Hove.

Renfrew, C.E. (1986) *Action Picture Test*, OUP, Oxford.

Renfrew, C.E. (1988) *Word-Finding Vocabulary Scale*, OUP, Oxford.

Reynell, J. and Huntley, M. (1993) *Reynell Developmental Language Scales*, 2nd edn, NFER-Nelson, Windsor.

Semel, E., Wiig, E.H. and Secord, W. (1994) *CELF-R UK (Clinical Evaluation of Language Fundamentals – Revised)*, The Psychological Corporation, London.

Snowling, M.J. (1980) The development of grapheme–phoneme correspondence in normal and dyslexic readers. *Journal of Experimental Psychology*, **29**, 294–305.

Vellutino, F.R. (1980) *Dyslexia: Theory and Research*, MIT Press, London.

Useful addresses

Drake Educational Associates (Language Master System)
St Fagans Road
Fairwater
Cardiff CF4 3AE

Scholastic Publications Ltd (Evan-Moor Books)
Westfield Road
Southam
Leamington Spa
Warks CV33 0JH

LDA
Duke Street
Wisbech
Cambridge PE13 2AE

Schofield and Sims Ltd
Dogley Hill
Fenay Bridge
Huddersfield HD8 0NQ

Taskmaster Ltd
Morris Road
Leicester LE2 6BR

Letterland Ltd
Barton
Cambridge CB3 7AY

4 The Occupational Therapist

Ingrid Linge

The Occupational Therapist, another relative newcomer in the field, is proving to be a vital link in the diagnosis and treatment of specific learning difficulties. It is becoming increasingly clear that not only do dyslexic children often benefit from the support of an Occupational Therapist, but dyspraxia frequently overlaps with the dyslexic syndrome. Without the subtlety of an Occupational Therapist's diagnostic input and considerable skills in the management of these dyspraxic difficulties, the progress of this particular group of children would be frustratingly slow. Ingrid Linge, Occupational Therapist at Fairley House, makes an enormous input into the children's capacity to be physically and organizationally available for learning.

P.G.

Introduction

The role of the Occupational Therapist is constantly being redefined. Originally concerned with the physical well-being of the adult population, it has been extended over the past decade to include children of all ages. There were always obvious advantages to addressing the congenital motor problems of the individual as early as possible. Referral was initially through the Health Service and was linked to the child's physical development. More recently, the educational implications of the difficulties diagnosed and treated by the Occupational Therapist have become apparent.

The disorders in children which might appropriately be addressed by the Occupational Therapist fall into four categories. The first is associated with visual, hearing or motor handicaps and include the problems of the blind, the deaf and those with neuro-motor problems such as are evident in cases of cerebral palsy. The second group includes children who have a mild, moderate or severe degree of learning disability. The third involves those children with environmental, cultural or economic disadvantages. Finally there are children with specific learning difficulties, whose handicap only affects their ability to function in certain closely defined areas.

Over the years more and more therapists came to realize that an important part of a child's daily life, i.e. the hours the child spends at school, was receiving very little therapeutic input. The current growth and specialization areas of the educational process, coupled with the ever-increasing knowledge in the field of psychology and physical and mental child development, made the eventual transition of occupational therapy services into the educational setting predictable. To cope with this transition, many Occupational Therapists started looking carefully at the developmental symptoms experienced by these children and their implications in acquiring the basic skills of literacy and numeracy. By combining medical findings with the status of the child's functional and educational skills, a specialist area has developed within the field of paediatric occupational therapy geared towards the diagnosing and management of the child with specific learning difficulties. Children of average to above average intelligence who are failing to achieve their educational potential because of problems of motor development or visual perception can now be diagnosed by an Occupational Therapist with experience in this specialist field. This development has depended on multidisciplinary cooperation in order to identify children who have normal measured intelligence, but cannot acquire certain well-defined academic skills such as reading, writing and numeracy. In the past these children could well have been labelled as underachievers, as emotionally disturbed or as having minimal brain dysfunction. As time has progressed, research in this field has produced more evidence on the nature of the difficulties experienced by these children and consensus as to the definition of a recognizable group of children with specific learning difficulties has been achieved.

Occupational Therapists are interested in how the child with specific learning difficulties performs in different situations. The child at school requires certain prerequisites for successful learning which include organization of the customary daily round of activities making up a routine part of normal school life. A learning problem can result from a child's brain being unable to organize sensory input or when the child's behaviour inhibits the learning process. A type of neural irregularity may be associated with difficulty in developing habits that support academic achievement, such as automatic use of verbal rehearsal when remembering a sequence of symbols, i.e. a telephone number, or the discipline required to do homework and study. The child may be unable to manage daily activities in ways that optimize this role performance.

Most often Occupational Therapists treat children with learning difficulties and sensory integrative disorders. They aim to improve efficiency of neural processing. While research shows that a sensory integrative approach benefits some children with learning difficulties, it is not appropriate for all.

Paediatric Occupational Therapists use a particular frame of reference which expands the neurobiological focus of development with reference to the sociocultural and environmental dimensions. Treatment cannot be offered in a vacuum but must be related to the everyday tasks confronting the child. Within this framework various different treatment approaches can be selected to suit the specific needs of the child. The focus of therapy is geared towards how effectively the child fulfils particular life roles in the family, school and community. Children in need of health care are nowadays seen as individuals who are required to meet specific expectations associated with particular roles. This assumption, when applied to the child with learning difficulties, translates into a concern over how well the child is performing in an educational setting, although their life outside school will also inevitably be affected by his problems and will benefit from intervention.

Assessments and tests

Within the specific time limitations of the assessment period, the Occupational Therapist will be looking at gross/fine motor coordination, visual perception, neurological and postural control and planning and organization of tasks. A specific battery of tests has been chosen to assess the above areas of functioning and this, together with general observation, is used for the specified diagnosis of learning difficulties. Through careful screening of each child the tests establish useful criteria for correct school placement. They also ensure that the child's remedial needs can be met through an appropriate individual education plan (IEP).

In order to assess gross/fine motor function the Movement ABC Test Battery has been developed (Henderson and Sugden, 1992). This test examines tasks involving manual dexterity, ball skills and balance reactions by age-related functional activities.

Visual perceptual skills are assessed using certain subtests of the Carrow Auditory–Visual Abilities Test (CAVAT) (Carrow-Woolfolk, 1981). The results provide a standardized percentile score of overall visual perceptual functioning and highlight areas of specific difficulty. Further investigation of visual motor integration skills is undertaken using the Beery Developmental Test of Visual–Motor Integration (Beery, 1982). This involves copying a series of geometric designs which become increasingly more complex. Analysis of these results gives an age-equivalent level of functioning and a standardized percentile score.

Investigation into visual–spatial perception is done by using the Jordan Left–Right Reversal Test (Jordan, 1980). This assesses the child's ability to recognize the correct orientation of letters and numbers.

A subsequent level of assessment involves the use of Jean Ayres' clinical observations. This assesses postural functioning, muscle tone, motor planning abilities, eye movements, laterality, bilateral integration and general gross motor coordination. Any neurological deficiencies and immature reflexes would also be revealed (Ayres, 1985).

At this stage assessment of the child's handwriting and pencil coordination will also take place.

It is not practical to administer all these tests during the time available on the assessment day and an appropriate selection must be made. However, if the child comes to Fairley House, it is possible to conduct further tests, as and when necessary, on site.

All the children at Fairley House School have been diagnosed as having specific learning difficulties. It is striking to observe how individuals present with different symptoms. Considering the complexity of the neural activity that enables learning, it is perhaps only reasonable to expect lack of complete homogeneity among learning-impaired children. In view of this, the importance of accurate diagnoses and individual management cannot be over-stressed. The following characteristics and views are now frequently used as a guide in identifying the child with a specific learning difficulty.

Most commonly seen is a wide discrepancy between academic achievement, ability and learning in a specific area, such as a discrepancy between what a child expresses verbally and what is expressed through their written work. Other apparently contradictory characteristics may be noted. This is reasonable, since not all possible symptoms will be present in one individual and indeed, it is likely that there will also be strengths in some specific areas. Specific learning difficulties can cover a broad spectrum and visual perceptual difficulties and motor problems may or may not form part of the pattern of difficulty. If the problems within the remit of the Occupational Therapist are present, they will almost certainly significantly affect the child's ability to perform. Areas of difficulty which concern the Occupational Therapist's functioning within the multidisciplinary team can be clearly defined.

- **Hyperactivity.** This is characterized by restlessness, which is often seen as an inability to sit still. This refers to excessive movement that may interfere with the child's ability to attend selectively to stimuli. The child appears to be in perpetual motion and mentally very 'butterfly minded'.
- **Hypoactivity.** This is the opposite of hyperactivity and refers to listlessness and sluggishness; it is not as common as hyperactivity.
- **Inattention.** This refers to the inability to focus attention on one task for any length of time.
- **Overattention.** This is the inability to break a focus after having been concentrating for a sustained period of time.
- **Motor difficulties.** Lack of coordination refers to the inability to move the muscles in a smooth manner. At a young age there may be signs of poor coordination or slow achievement of developmental milestones. For example, the child may have difficulty throwing a ball, skipping or running. The child may appear to be clumsy and trip frequently. Low muscle tone may affect the child's postural stability, which could contribute to the difficulties some children experience with maintaining a stable seated position required for most academic tasks.
- **Perceptual disorders.** These are most frequently seen in visual, auditory, tactile, proprioceptive and vestibular perception. Problems in olfactory and gustatory perception are less likely to be associated with a learning difficulty. Visual–spatial problems may interfere with accurate copying of letters. Children with auditory perceptual dysfunction may have difficulty distinguishing the ringing of a telephone from that of a doorbell. Tactile, proprioceptive and vestibular perception will be discussed below.
- **Perseveration.** The central element in perseveration is that the child will repeat an action. An everyday analogy of this behaviour would be a gramophone record getting stuck whilst playing. This can occur over several behavioural domains, such as repetition of certain phrases in speech, but is more frequently seen in writing. An example would be if the child were writing the word 'dog', he would be continually repeating the 'o' pattern and thus never completing the word with the 'g'.
- **Disorders in information processing.** The central aspect of this disorder is that the child will be unable to connect the written symbol or the letter with the sound of that letter when spoken and therefore will reproduce incorrect letters when writing and spelling. Another aspect of this problem is that the child will confuse letters which have the same symbol orientated in a different fashion, for example 'b' and 'd', and therefore reproduce the incorrect letter for a requested word when spelling.

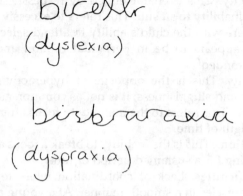

Fig. 4.1 An example of b/d reversal.

The remediation of these symptoms is best approached through an understanding of the sensory motor systems of the individual. The brain translates sensory impulses into meaningful information and organizes an appropriate motor response. If the brain is to function at an optimum level it must both receive and integrate a constant stream of stimuli, especially from the body. If this is done ineffectively, our ability to cope with the world diminishes. Learning is a function of the brain and learning difficulties are assumed to reflect some deviation in neural function. The theory is that disordered sensory integration accounts for some aspects of learning difficulties and that enhancing sensory integration will make learning easier. A sensory integrative approach differs from many other procedures in that it does not teach specific skills, such as matching visual stimuli, drawing lines from one point to another or learning to remember a sequence of sounds. Rather the objective is to enhance the brain's ability to learn effective methods of processing sensory information. If the brain develops the capacity to perceive, remember and motor plan, the ability can be applied to the mastery of a broad spectrum of tasks, including academic skills, regardless of the specific content. If the integrative process is not occurring properly, the result is a disruption in learning, in performance and in the pattern of life as we know it.

If we look closely at the process of sensory integration, we can see a sequence of stages evolving, each one distinct but interdependent. There are seven major sensory systems in the human body, not all of which will be familiar to the non-specialist. These systems are responsible for providing the brain with the necessary information regarding the environment and the state of the body within it. This information is vital if the brain is to produce the appropriate response that would enable the individual to interact successfully and learn from the environment. The visual and auditory systems are easily recognized, as is the tactile system which is responsible for touch sensation. The olfactory and gustatory systems are responsible for the sensations of smell and taste and do not form an integral part of the process involved with learning. The vestibular system is responsible for the information picked up by receptors situated in the inner ear which react to changes in the position of the head in relation to gravity and form an integral part of the body's motor system. The proprioceptive system picks up information from receptors within the muscles and joints of the body and relays vital information to the brain with regard to the body's positioning within the environment. Closely associated with the proprioceptive system is the kinaesthetic sense. This is the term used to describe the sensation of the body moving through space.

Research (Ayres, 1966, 1969) has postulated that the tactile system is a major source of sensory input which helps build the body scheme or concept of the body needed for motor planning. The vestibular system orientates the body in space and as it moves through space. This, in combination with the proprioceptive system, is considered to be of major importance as its mechanisms are intricately linked with the development of muscle tone, the control of eye movements, visual and auditory perception and coordination skills, as well as automatic functions such as heart rate, respiration and emotions. In the developmental process, in order to reach an upright posture, stand and ultimately walk, primitive postural reflexes which are present from birth need to be inhibited and replaced by voluntary motor control. If certain reflexes are not inhibited and integrated, they will affect the normal path of motor development and certain patterns of motor actions may predominate, resulting in poor posture, impaired body movements and coordination, plus immature balance and equilibrium reactions. It is reasonable to conclude that people suffering from this lack of integration would be hesitant to perform any motor actions which threaten the state of equilibrium which the person is finding so difficult to achieve.

Doctor Jean Ayres was an Occupational Therapist who was the first therapist to research and develop the theory and practice of sensory integration. Dr Ayres, from her practice as an Occupational Therapist, was aware that defined activities used with children had broader implications in promoting increased independence in life skills. She felt that the main reason for this was the way the activities were used with children, which somehow established a sensory motor pattern leading to the interpretation of sensory input signals. The development of these sensory motor patterns enhanced the brain's ability to learn how to master tasks regardless of specific content. In other words, perhaps merely teaching a child to put their clothes on in a repetitive order does not enhance motor patterns and therefore the task is not mastered indefinitely. The child must give cognitive meaning to that pattern of movement, which will result in the transfer of skills to a number of similar tasks. Without verifying every aspect of the theory, it is possible to state that the practical recommendations seem to produce positive results in many cases.

In considering the child diagnosed as having a specific learning difficulty, it is important to discuss the components of the disorder that would best be addressed by an Occupational Therapist. A definition of dyspraxia will be discussed below, as well as a description of the manifestations of dyspraxia and how best to address them. As a symptom of dyspraxia and because problems in this area are commonly associated with specific learning disabilities, the acquisition of handwriting skills and strategies for remediating their dysfunction are given considerable attention.

Dyspraxia

Praxis is defined as the ability of the brain to conceive of, organize and carry out a sequence of unfamiliar actions. This is commonly known as motor planning. Dr Ayres (1985) defined dyspraxia as a motor planning disorder and as a disorder of sensory integration interfering with the ability to plan and execute skilled motor tasks. Many people refer to these symptoms as 'the clumsy child syndrome'.

When assessing the factors involved in carrying out skilled motor actions three processes can be identified.

* Ideation or conceptualization (grasping the idea of how the body can use objects in the physical environment or producing the idea of an action).
* Planning a scheme of action.
* The motor execution.

These three processes are common to all facets or manifestations of dyspraxia. To illustrate these processes, a child may come into a room and see a scooter board on the floor. If he ignores the object it may be because there is no ability to conceptualize the use of the scooter board and if this facility is lacking then the response will not be that of normal children who are immediately responsive to a scooter board. The child might lack the planning skills necessary to make use of the board. If the child attempts to imitate the therapist, who models one way of using the board, he is demonstrating his ability to plan a course of action. The result of the scooter board being an unfamiliar object is that the child has had to plan unusual movements. The degree and accuracy with which these movements are planned will be clear from their execution. Implications can be drawn from a child's methods and measure of success.

There are times when a standardized test cannot be used to assess a child. The child's interaction in a therapist-guided activity can be used as a diagnostic alternative to make a professional judgement. It is at these times that the child's innate drive to engage in purposeful activity can be observed. When the drive for interaction with the physical world is there, but purposefulness, success or adaptive skill is inadequate, then the problem may be dyspraxia. Analysing how the child plays can reveal a great deal. If the child's imagination is expressed more in verbal and fanciful ways than in object manipulation or environmental interaction, the child may be dyspraxic. If the child simply pushes a toy instead of engaging in more complex body movement, both conceptualization and planning may be poor.

The great advantage of a school environment in which to conduct an assessment is that the child's coordination and, indeed, behaviour can also be observed during playtime in the park, not to mention games and PE classes.

The first of the three processes, ideation, is a term commonly used by Occupational Therapists and is similar in meaning to conceptualization. It is a thinking process. An example of ideation in everyday life would be a child recognizing his desire to drink a glass of milk. Ideation would be the process by which the child would think through the actions to achieve this goal. In a normal child this process is in most cases automatic. Only complex tasks might cause the child to dwell on this aspect in achieving a goal. However, a young dyspraxic child would find this element a major obstacle in planning how to achieve simple goals, for example how to play with equipment and toys. This situation is exacerbated as most dyspraxic children have limited manual manipulation skills. Nevertheless, being young and full of natural drive to be active, these children are often very active in a non-purposeful way. As noted earlier, hyperactivity often accompanies dyspraxia. Parents of dyspraxic children often report they are difficult to live with. Dr Ayres postulated that ideation was perhaps the very first step in the development of the ability to organize behaviour relative to the physical environment.

As already mentioned, ideation is a cognitive approach, one that is dependent on sensory integration and resultant knowledge of available body actions. Additional intellectual processes, including knowledge of objects and their potential use, develop out of use of the body in purposeful activity with those objects. The dyspraxic child is most likely to have trouble choosing an appropriate activity and utilizing equipment appropriately, such as putting a track together to make a railway or even simply piling large bricks on top of each other to make a tower. Later, parents often complain of the difficulty in getting a child off to school. This may be merely a later manifestation of this same motor planning difficulty. A common facet of these problems is the difficulty in forming an idea or conceptualizing the plan of action. The end product cannot be be anticipated easily and visualizing the necessary intervening stages appears to be difficult.

The second of the three processes, planning a scheme of action, involves the motor plan. This is a consciously formulated, internal plan of action which occurs before actual motor execution. Motor or action planning is the in-between process which bridges ideation and motor execution to enable adaptive interaction with the physical world. Adaptive interaction can be defined as the ability to react appropriately to different physical stimuli to produce calculated results. Planning requires thinking. If one has to think about actions, motor planning is probably occurring. If one does not have to think about them, the actions have probably become automatic and no longer require planning. For example, consider yourself as a child and recall the effort and concentration required when first learning how to ride a bicycle. In retrospect it is difficult to visualize yourself in that position when each step involved in the carrying out of the action had to be explicitly defined and understood, both in thought and in action, before the entire process of balancing, pedalling and moving on the bicycle was mastered to become the natural, automatic process that we experience today.

The steps involved in learning to carry out a motor action such as riding a bicycle can just as easily be likened to the cognitive process involved in learning to read. Initially, an extreme amount of energy and effort is required on the part of the child in attempting to decipher and understand the symbols used to relay meaningful information in the form of the written word. These initial stages require a great deal of time and practice before the process can become automatic. Both the motor and the cognitive actions required in the examples cited above needed effective motor planning to ensure success in the adaptive response produced in learning to ride a bicycle and to read. If a child is thinking about a plan of action it is best not to distract him through irrelevant verbal messages but rather to provide simple instructions such as 'Put your foot here' or 'It sounds similar to ...' that may prompt the child a little further along the planning process. Therapy is designed to promote planning and thus activities requiring thinking are used as a basis of treatment for children with dyspraxia.

The brain must have various kinds of information to enable it to motor plan. First, it must have the idea of the purposeful act. It must be able to conceptualize the action and its goal. Then it must know how the body is designed and how it functions as a mechanical being. This information comes from the tactile, proprioceptive, kinaesthetic and vestibular systems. Vision and hearing also help. The motor plan is made up of a series of different movements which must be ordered into a smoothly executed, composite, whole act. This involves sequencing the movements which in turn consists of a change in position or movement in relation to total performance. A sequencing problem may lie in either making the change from one position to another or in remembering or knowing the order in which the movement should be executed. With dyspraxic children the most evident lack of sequencing ability is seen when a task requires more than one clearly defined action which would normally be accomplished in one continuous movement. For example, a child may ride a scooter board down a ramp heading towards a soft tower of blocks to knock down but stop just before reaching the blocks, then proceed to knock down the blocks as a separate plan of action. Timing is important in the sequencing of actions during purposeful activity. A timing disorder may be seen in the child who has difficulty letting go of a trapeze from which he is swinging. Some children cannot release at a time appropriate for falling onto a mat or cushion and will return to an earlier position before letting go. Some dyspraxic children will strike at a swinging or hanging ball a split second too late.

Whereas ideation and motor planning create the problems described, the final stage of the praxis act, execution, is not likely to be a major source of difficulty in children with dyspraxia. However, it is

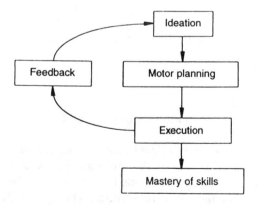

Fig. 4.2 Diagrammatic representation of the feedback continuum postulated by Ayres to explain the theory of praxis.

only in the ultimate execution of the act that the quality of ideation and motor planning are revealed. This process is part of a continuum whereby execution is followed by sensory feedback before starting the cycle again (Fig. 4.2). While dyspraxic execution may be clumsy, dyspraxic children usually have close to normal neuromotor skills. Ideation and planning distinguish praxis from a purely motor function.

MANIFESTATIONS OF DYSPRAXIA

The Occupational Therapist identifies dyspraxia when poor motor planning interferes with large body actions observed when a child attempts a gross motor task. It is suggested that the dyspraxia manifested in this manner could be defined as 'postural dyspraxia' (Ayres, 1985), as opposed to 'constructional dyspraxia' which will be defined later. A disorder of postural dyspraxia is most easily identified in motor clumsiness, including difficulty with or lack of enjoyment of sports, learning to dress oneself, craftwork expected in nursery and primary classrooms, use of cutlery at the table and handwriting. Testing of children for postural dyspraxia involves movements of the entire body and not simply the use of both arms, which is described as bilateral integration. In testing, children are expected to imitate movement actions with little verbal help so as not to provide auditory input that may assist with the processing of the motor plan. Whole body movements sometimes require considerable mid-line muscle function, as in rotating the trunk, bending the head forward, walking backwards or rolling over. Several tasks have been selected as being most suitable for identifying dyspraxia. They reflect postural as well as manual functions. These tasks were developed by Gubbay (1978) and consist of the following.

- Throwing a tennis ball into the air and clapping hands before catching it.
- Rolling a tennis ball underfoot in a zigzag fashion between matchboxes.
- Threading beads.
- Inserting shaped objects into appropriate slots.

Constructional dyspraxia relates more to the inability to relate the concrete part to the whole, as in assembling a jigsaw. It can be assessed by administering a design copy test, such as the Beery Developmental Test of Visual–Motor Integration (Beery, 1982), as well as giving the child an actual three-dimensional object manipulation task, such as the object assembly in the Wechsler Intelligence Scale for

Children III (Wechsler, 1991). Both these methods involve combining elements into an entity which is more than just the sum of its parts. The brain, through directing motor behaviour which acts directly on the physical environment, whether it be pencil or blocks, creates an object by uniting a number of parts into a coherent whole. Constructional dyspraxia, while dependent upon motor processes for execution, is less a motor problem than an inability to conceptualize either the finished product or the steps involved in its realization or the relationship of the parts used to create the whole. It is heavily dependent on visual space perception. Construction of - three-dimensional objects does provide both a visible and concrete demonstration of a dyspraxic child's inability to manipulate objects in space.

Writing, spelling and numeracy can all be affected, since all these skills involve a sequential series of actions to build up a meaningful end product from a series of intermediate stages.

MANAGEMENT OF DYSPRAXIA

The analysis of these three processes helps to determine appropriate intervention. Emphasis will normally be on the first two processes, since once these are mastered, execution will probably occur naturally.

Ideation is the first process that needs to be addressed. If the child does not have adequate ideation, they will not have the ability to focus on an appropriate task and will probably show little interaction with the immediate environment. In this case the therapist needs to help the child by having suitable activities previously prepared and preferably modelling the appropriate actions in order to convey the idea. The selected activities should offer both challenge and success. If the child is only partially successful, the therapist should help the child to be completely successful. If the child leaves a task with a feeling of failure, he will probably not return to it. An example of this would be when a child becomes frustrated with doing a fine motor task, such as threading small beads onto a string; because he was not able to do the activity successfully, the activity will most likely be abandoned and not attempted again. This is often the case with many nursery children who, once they have failed to successfully complete a fine motor task, will actively avoid spontaneous participation in similar activities.

After the child has grasped the idea of what is to be done, he must plan a course of action to implement the idea. The central concepts under consideration when arranging an activity for planning are the sensory input demands of the activity. For this process to be successful, the child needs to have adequate knowledge of his body and how to use it effectively in interactions with the environment. Treatment of dyspraxia usually starts by addressing postural dyspraxia and this is most effective when the therapy involves whole body actions, which generate the greatest amount of sensory input from the body. Activities should therefore be chosen with the child's specific vestibular, tactile and proprioceptive needs in mind.

An example of an activity suitable for addressing postural dyspraxia would be a game using a large physio ball, whereby the child could be asked to get himself over the ball without the help of any other equipment. The various positions the child assumes in accomplishing this task would fulfil the sensory demands needed in dealing with their postural dyspraxia. The physical properties of the ball provide the vestibular input and the large body surface in contact with the ball provides the tactile input. The pushing and pulling involved in preparing to launch the body onto the ball and when landing on the other side would fulfil the proprioceptive demands of the body. While these sources of input are normally generated during a well-chosen activity, occasionally direct application through passive means is appropriate. For example, brushing a child's hands with a non-scratch brush prior to engaging in a fine motor activity would provide the tactile input needed to assist with the planning of the motor actions required for the activity.

Dyspraxic children often have poorly developed basic whole body motor patterns such as total flexion. For example, bringing the head to touch the knees while lying on the back; total extension, which involves lifting the head, arms and legs off the floor while lying on the stomach, rotation; which is seen when turning the body around to see behind while sitting on a chair, and gross diagonal rotatory patterns which are observed when picking up an item from the floor using both hands while sitting on a chair. Visual direction of body action is often poor in dyspraxic children and is another indication of poor sensory integration. Often children must be reminded to look at what they are doing and where they are going.

Once therapeutic attention has been directed successfully to ideation and planning demands, execution of a practical task will probably be performed without much difficulty.

In summary, then, it is best to begin treating a dyspraxic child at as young an age as possible, preferably before the age of three years. The inner drive to be active wanes at the age of seven or eight, as does the potential to develop praxis. Activities used can provide the necessary sensory input from the body and eyes. Sometimes the sensory input is provided by the therapist. Available activities need to fit the child's ideation and planning ability and the Occupational Therapist helps the child's performance and development in both areas. Activities must challenge the child but also ensure success, perhaps with the therapist's help, but the child must make the effort. Success must be the reward. Treating dyspraxic children requires a highly specialized, skilled and creative Occupational Therapist.

Handwriting

ASSESSMENT

In the school setting, once children have been identified as having poor handwriting, a full assessment needs to be carried out to identify the reasons for their difficulties, which are often specific to the individual. Information needs to be gathered from as many sources as possible to develop an understanding of the child's neuromotor development, cognitive and psychosocial behaviour, environmental factors and skill acquisition which could all contribute to the child's failure to produce legible handwriting.

Skilled observation of the child writing in the classroom is mandatory in the information-gathering process. In these situations it is important to consider the child's behaviour and whether or not the child can attend to the task of writing independently. Other concerns address the child's distractibility – visual or auditory – and the child's level of frustration with writing. During the observation, the level of difficulty of the writing tasks should also be noted. For example, a writing task of composing a sentence requires different sensorimotor and cognitive skills from taking dictation or copying a sentence. The classroom environment, the child's actual physical placement in the class and their interaction with the teacher and peers also give more information. Discussion with the child's teacher is another useful way of gathering data. The teacher often describes how the child's performance in writing and other subjects affects the child in the classroom situation.

A specific handwriting policy has been adopted by Fairley House School and forms part of the whole school philosophy in teaching handwriting. The school has developed an easy-to-read handwriting script which closely resembles the script seen in reading books. The letters are grouped into families according to common patterns used in their formation (Fig. 4.3). The children are taught cursive writing from the start, as the process of joining letters in a word assists them with understanding and conceptualizing the word patterns needed in spelling.

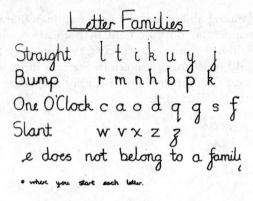

Letter Families

Straight   l t i k u y j
Bump   r m n h b p k
One O'Clock c a o d q g s f
Slant   w v x z z
e does not belong to a family

• where you start each letter.

Fig. 4.3 Letters of the alphabet grouped into families according to letter formation patterns.

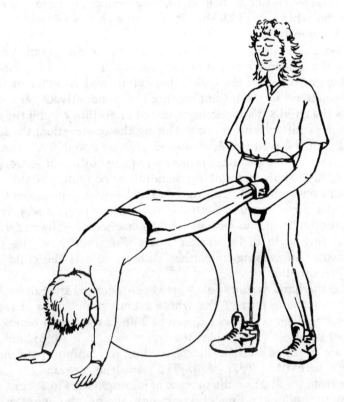

Fig. 4.4 The use of the therapy ball for shoulder joint stability.

When evaluating the child's sensorimotor foundations, it is important to examine the neuromuscular mechanisms contributing to the development of postural control, shoulder stability and muscle tone. Postural control is the base from which purposeful movement can occur. Frequently, children lacking a stable trunk and experiencing variations and fluctuations in muscle tone demonstrate poor handwriting. They are unable to sustain an upright position or make the needed postural adjustments while focusing on fine motor activities, such as handwriting. Another neuromuscular requisite, shoulder stability, may be affected by variations in muscle tone, an inability to co-contract the various muscle groups around the joints and a lack of fluidity of shoulder blade movements (Fig. 4.4). Without the stabilization of the shoulder, elbow and wrist, the speed and dexterity of the hand's intrinsic movements when manipulating the writing tool become impeded and inefficient neuromuscular mechanisms commonly interfere with legible handwriting.

The areas of sensory integrative functioning most directly related to handwriting encompass the tactile, proprioceptive and visual systems, kinaesthesia, visual perception and motor planning. The tactile and proprioceptive systems provide information to the child regarding the grasp of the pencil and rubber and the stabilization of the paper. To write well, a child must be able to maintain the position of his head and eyes relative to the writing task. In addition, the child must be able to perform the rather complex set of optical skills needed for reading. This includes saccadic eye movements, which involve the concurrent activity of 'sampling' the text before and after the word or phrase being focused on. This prepares the mind to receive the data on the written page and is essential for good reading skills. Writing complicates this task, where the child not only has to cope with holding the train of thought being transcribed on the paper, but needs to focus on the pencil actually forming the letters.

The amount of pressure a child applies to the writing tool and the paper, the ability to write within parameters and the directionality of the implement is termed 'kinaesthesia', i.e. an awareness of the extent, weight and direction of movement. Children with kinaesthetic dysfunction may press too hard or not hard enough with their pencil while writing and may be confused when trying to direct their writing tools to form letters or to write between lines. Visual perception, the ability to organize and interpret what is seen, affects handwriting chiefly in two areas. Positioning space or the ability to determine the spatial relationship of figures and objects to self or other forms and objects (McGourty *et al.*, 1989) affects the child's ability to space between the letters of a word and words of a sentence and to place letters correctly on a horizontal line. When writing, children with a poor understanding of position in space may demonstrate underspacing (running together or overlapping letters and words), overspacing (leaving large spaces between letters and words) and improper placement of letters on the writing line. Form constancy, the capacity to recognize forms and objects as the same in various environments, positions and sizes (Mcgourty *et al.*, 1989), allows the child to discriminate between letters and numerals that are very similar such as b/d, p/q, 2/5, which is critical for writing. The lack of form constancy may result in reversal of letters and transposition of words. Finally, motor planning in writing influences the child's ability to plan, sequence and execute the letter forms and the ordering of letters to build words.

Motor aspects related to handwriting involve activity tolerance, bilateral integration, visual motor integration and fine motor coordination. Obviously activity tolerance, sustaining a writing activity for a length of time, is needed in order for the child to practise and master the skill. Both strength and endurance are needed to persist in a handwriting task for an extended period of time. Bilateral integration includes both symmetrical and asymmetrical movements of the body needed for an activity (Exner, 1989). Writing consists mainly of asymmetrical movements. For example, stabilizing the paper with the non-preferred hand while holding the pencil with the preferred hand may not be achieved when children have difficulties dissociating movement of the upper extremities. Visual motor integration, the ability to coordinate visual information with a motor response, allows a child to reproduce letters and numbers required for acquiring literacy and numeracy skills. According to Exner (1989), three aspects of fine motor control which affect handwriting are:

- isolation of movements;
- grading of movements;
- timing of movements.

An inability to isolate and grade hand and finger movements may result in inadequate pencil grasp and poor skills in other areas which demand similar gradation of movement. To expand on this ability to grade movement, in order to write children must be able to control the amount of pressure plus the amount of movement required to form the pattern of a particular letter. For example, a child who can write well, if asked to write an 'o', would show a symbol of even thickness and symmetry in performing the task, and only the fingers would move. When asked to write a series of letters, such as in spelling a word, a child with good grading would write it in a smooth, flowing manner. In addition the child may bring either his forearm, elbow or shoulder into action when producing large quantities of work. Children demonstrating poor grading of muscles usually use compensatory techniques to stabilize their pencils, most frequently observed as fingers locked into extension or fisted into flexion. Timing affects the rhythm and flow of writing and inadequacies are exhibited by the child as slow, laboured, jerky writing or rapid, haphazard handwriting skills. Fine motor control includes in-hand manipulation, described by Exner (1989) as the 'process of adjusting objects within the hand after grasp'; for example, when picking up a coin from a surface and transferring the coin to the palm of the hand. As explained by Exner (1992), after grasping a pencil, 'shifting' (the linear movement of the pencil among the fingers needed to adjust it for writing) and 'rotating' (the movement of the pencil around an axis) are essential for vertically turning the pencil from grasp to placement for writing or erasing.

As part of the handwriting assessment, the child's attention span, information processing using the visual, verbal and motor channels, sequencing and conceptual skills all need to be considered to understand the overall picture of the child presenting with a handwriting dysfunction. These factors, together with the child's self-concept, interests, behaviour and motivation, affect their performance of handwriting. Often, children with poor handwriting develop low self-esteem. Each time the child writes in a sloppy, haphazard manner, it looks right back up at them and states 'This is a mess'. For the child, this message is a constant reminder of failure at school, diminishing an already fragile self-esteem. From this poor self-concept, low motivation for handwriting may result.

At Fairley House School informal tests are used to assess children's handwriting. Aspects of handwriting such as legibility components, speed of writing and ergonomics are all factors carefully considered. It is of crucial importance that the size of chairs, the adjustment of the desk or writing surface and the body posture of the child are all monitored by the Occupational Therapist to achieve optimal control. Handwriting tasks similar to those required of the pupil in the classroom are used as part of the assessment, including dictation, far and near-point copying, upper and lower case letter writing, composition and endurance.

Dictation is the writing of letters or words when verbally requested by the assessor and emphasizes the child's ability to make a motor response to auditory directions. This skill is particularly important when spelling words. Copying is reproducing letters, numbers and words from a presented sample of either cursive or non-cursive writing. Frequently, copying tasks occur in the classroom as children copy mathematical problems from text books and as they reproduce a sentence copied from the whiteboard while seated at their desks. Far-point copying entails copying from a distant vertical board to the horizontal writing surface, whereas near-point copying is duplicating letters or words from a nearby horizontal surface, usually on the same page or at least on the same writing surface. Writing the alphabet in both upper and lower cases involves the child's sequencing of the alphabet, the consistency of letter case and the formation of each individual letter. Composition of a sentence or paragraph is seen in the way children compose their stories and poems in the classroom situation.

When examining a child's handwriting, the first question commonly asked is 'Is it legible?' Legibility is defined in terms of letter formation, alignment, spacing, sizing and slant. Any one of these components may affect the readability of a sample of handwriting, but when two or more components are combined, the legibility of the handwriting sample may be seriously affected.

Alston and Taylor (1987) identified several factors contributing to handwriting illegibility in primary school-aged children. When considering letter formation they identified the following common characteristics:

- incorrect letter formation;
- inadequate start and finish positions when forming letters;
- poor rounding of the letters;
- incomplete letter closure;
- inadequate letter ascenders and descenders.

Alignment refers to the placement of the letter on the writing line with the ability to write on lines of appropriate width for age expectations. All children at Fairley House School are initially started on multi-lined paper and as the alignment and sizing of their letters become more consistent, they are gradually weaned onto ordinary lined paper.

Spacing refers to the way letters are distributed within the words and how words are spaced within sentences. Uniformity of spacing is considered an essential key in producing legible writing. Determining if letters are similar in size and if the size of writing is appropriate also contributes to legibility. Although difficult to measure objectively, slant should be consistent and when it is not uniform it makes handwriting difficult to read, even when other components of legibility are intact (Fig. 4.5).

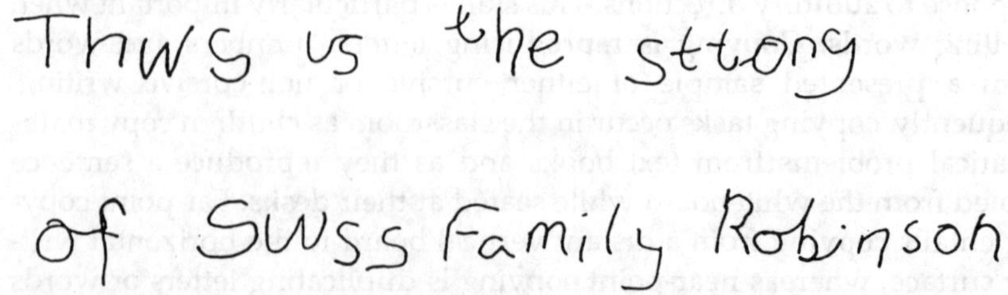

Thws vs the sttong

of SWss Family Robinson

Fig. 4.5 Samples of children's handwriting demonstrating poor legibility.

When assessing handwriting speed, no standardized results have yet been published on the norm for the number of letters produced per minute for school-aged children. Despite this lack of objective data, for pupils to accomplish an acceptable amount of work in the classroom, a certain writing speed must be maintained. The speed and level of skill in writing may deteriorate when the complexity or volume of the writing task increases or the speed demanded is faster than the child's natural speed of writing. It is important, therefore, for the therapist and the teacher to determine if the child's written productivity is adequate for the time constraints and the volume of work involved.

Endurance is observed in the assessment session or in the classroom situation while the child writes five or six sentences. Children with poor handwriting frequently cannot sustain the legibility of their writing as the length of the task increases. As the child tires, letter sizes may become smaller, writing more laboured and letters or words omitted. When endurance is poor and the child's writing pace is slow, he does not have the opportunities to practice letter formation as do other children.

As children are engaged in the writing process, ergonomic factors such as posture, upper body stability and mobility and pencil grasp are all observed and documented and their posture is analysed. Does the child support his head when writing or lay the head on the desktop? Does the child kneel on the chair in an effort to gain more proprioceptive input through the arms and legs? Are the chair and the desk at the appropriate heights for writing in the classroom? Stability and mobility of the upper body refers to the stabilization of the shoulder, elbow and wrist to allow for the mobility of the hand to manipulate the writing implement. What is the position of the writing arm? What other parts of the body are moving during writing? Does the assisting hand steady the writing paper? Is the writing movement smooth or jerky?

Finally, the primary ergonomic focus for most Occupational Therapists is pencil grasp. How does the child hold the pencil? What amount of pressure is used on the pencil? When directed, can the child adjust the pencil in his hand? The dynamic tripod grasp involves resting the writing implement on the middle finger and controlling it with the pads of the thumb and index fingers. This is typically the grip most Occupational Therapists and teachers encourage when writing (Fig. 4.6), but variations are often seen amongst children and adults without a handwriting dysfunction. Because of the increased incidence of the lateral tripod grip (Fig. 4.7) amongst children and adults with no handwriting problems, this grip is now regarded as being an appropriate alternative to the dynamic tripod grasp when writing.

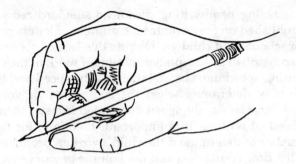

Fig. 4.6 Diagram showing the dynamic tripod grip.

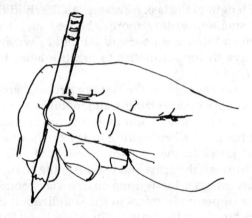

Fig. 4.7 Illustration of the lateral tripod grip.

MANAGEMENT OF HANDWRITING DYSFUNCTION

From a traditional, educational model, occupational therapy intervention for a child with a handwriting dysfunction may appear unusual.
However, Occupational Therapists can use a variety of therapeutic
approaches for the remediation of handwriting problems. Theoretical
approaches which apply to handwriting intervention include:

- neuromuscular
- acquisitional
- multisensory
- biomechanical
- motivational.

Developing and implementing effective and comprehensive hand-writing intervention programmes for children requires attention to all aspects of handwriting. Integrating the neuromuscular, acquisitional, multisensory, biomechanical and motivational approaches challenges the Occupational Therapist's expertise in devising a creative and exciting intervention unique for each child with handwriting difficulties. It is important when considering any intervention plan for handwriting that a balance between these five approaches is kept in mind. At certain times in a remedial session, one approach may predominate in the therapist's attempts to assist the child in experiencing a greater variety of avenues for learning and thus increase the opportunities for the child to master handwriting.

Neuromuscular approach

Postural preparation for writing originates from this theory. Preparing children's bodies and upper extremities to write is critical in any type of handwriting intervention programme, whether delivered in a group setting or in an individual session with the child. An intervention programme using this approach is particularly effective with a child identified as experiencing movement difficulties due to an imbalance in muscle tone. When utilizing this approach the following three strategies are recommended:

- modulating muscle tone throughout the trunk and upper extremities;
- ensuring free movement of the shoulder joint;
- promoting proximal stability.

Modulating muscle tone throughout the trunk and upper extremities may consist of increasing, decreasing or balancing tone. Increasing tone in children may be achieved by activities such as jumping jacks, obstacle courses that include pulling on a rope or fast foot manoeuvring in between the rungs of a ladder placed on the floor, or lifting or pushing furniture. For children whose muscle tone needs to be decreased, slow movements involving rolling and rocking provide inhibitory inputs necessary to achieve this. In the classroom, a child's postural tone may be reduced prior to writing by gently rocking in time to slow rhythmical music. Balancing muscle tone can be achieved through active weight shifting in a half-kneel stance or bending sideways to the left and right in sitting.

In individual sessions, the Occupational Therapist can prepare the child posturally for writing by ensuring free movement of the child's shoulder. This will often involve hands-on contact by the therapist to facilitate this smooth movement. Activities involving weightbearing, compression and traction are all useful in facilitating smooth scapular movements of the shoulder. In the classroom, useful activities to promote smooth scapular movements involve having the seated child holding their hands straight in front of them, with the backs of the hands together, making slow, circular arm motions or having the seated child, with hands on opposite shoulders, lift his elbows up and back down slowly.

Frequently, children with handwriting dysfunction experience poor proximal joint stability. To encourage muscular stability of the neck, shoulders, elbows and wrists, games such as animal walks which involve weight bearing on the upper extremities (bear walk, creeping worm or frog jumps) are beneficial in promoting proximal stability.

When needed, postural preparation must be the preliminary component of handwriting intervention and should occur in a 5-minute period before the instructional writing programme begins.

Acquisitional approach

In any handwriting intervention, a sequenced, instructional programme is required to enable the child to acquire and master handwriting proficiency. This skill, like any other acquisitional skill, can be improved through practice, repetition, feedback and reinforcement.

Certain principles are essential in ensuring an effective and successful handwriting programme. These include handwriting being taught directly and not incidentally and implemented in short daily lessons with letters being introduced in sequential progression. Handwriting should also be 'overlearned' and applied in a meaningful context for the child. The handwriting programme should build on mastered letters and those being learned, excluding any letters the child does not know or is forming improperly. Practising letters incorrectly strengthens unwelcome perceptual–motor patterns in the child who needs no more reinforcing of poor handwriting.

As soon as two or three letters are introduced and mastered, the child can then begin to put them in a meaningful context, namely words. For example, if a child had only learned the lower case letters 'a' and 'd', he could write two words, 'add' and 'dad'. During each intervention period, newly learned letters are joined with previously mastered ones to form words. This immediate reinforcement of writing words is much more purposeful and powerful for the child than writing a string of repeated letters.

Numerous reviews (Bergman and McLaughlin, 1988; Peck, Askov and Fairchild, 1980) on remediating strategies and modes of instruction in teaching handwriting indicate that a combination of techniques seem more desirable and effective than any one method. The following instructional approach sequentially blends modelling, tracing, stimulus fading, copying, composing, self-monitoring and peer recording.

- Modelling involves the therapist naming the letter to be written and making the letter on a lined writing surface while verbally cueing the child. The therapist not only models the letter but also the action to write the letter, repeating it two or three times.
- The child then traces over the letter as the therapist repeats the verbal cues and, if needed, provides visual cues also.
- Stimulus fading occurs when the child can successfully form the letters requiring less verbal and visual cueing as the process of forming the letters is learned.
- Although some children can imitate a letter correctly after modelling, those with perceptual–motor deficits may require both tracing and stimulus fading in order to reach the copying phase. When copying, the child does not observe the therapist producing the letter but only the end product and then attempts to reproduce it. Children should copy the learned letter until formation is acceptable to the therapist and the child. Once mastery of the letter is achieved, the child can begin copying words that include the learned letter and previously mastered letters.
- Following successful copying, the therapist may dictate words and the spelling of the words for the child to write.
- Children should then be given the opportunity to compose their own words which include mastered letters. Subsequently they will be encouraged to create their own sentences.
- Self-monitoring requires each child to become more actively involved in the handwriting programme by assuming responsibility for correcting his own work. With younger children, self-correction may occur verbally to analyse letter formation and overall legibility, whereas the older child may follow a checklist to examine written work (Fig. 4.8).
- When instructing a group of children, peer recording is an influential tool, especially when children are unable to be objective in self-correcting. By evaluating a peer's handwriting, children are able to be more objective in analysing and marking accuracies and faults and then they can apply similar standards to their own written work. In this process it is important for the therapist to model positive reinforcement by noting good writing as well as errors.

How do I Write? Checklist

NAME   DATE

I sit in the proper position.	Yes ( )	No ( )
My paper is at the right angle.	Yes ( )	No ( )
I hold my pencil the correct way.	Yes ( )	No ( )
I use a pencil grip.	Yes ( )	No ( )
My letters are properly formed.	Yes ( )	No ( )
My letters are the same size.	Yes ( )	No ( )
My letters with tails are of equal length.	Yes ( )	No ( )
My tall letters are the same height.	Yes ( )	No ( )
I write properly on the line.	Yes ( )	No ( )
My letters are on the same slant.	Yes ( )	No ( )
The spacing between my words is even.	Yes ( )	No ( )
My letters are joined correctly.	Yes ( )	No ( )
I use capital letters correctly.	Yes ( )	No ( )
I use full stops correctly.	Yes ( )	No ( )

I need to work on:

1.

2.

3.

Fig. 4.8   Sample of a student self-evaluation handwriting checklist.

When learning proper letter formation other components of legibility, namely size, slant and alignment, are addressed inherently; spacing and speed are not. Overspacing and underspacing between words are common among children who have perceptual problems. For these children, spacing can be demonstrated by using actual objects to represent the space between words, e.g. the width of a pencil shaft or finger spaces using the forefinger. The object can later be imagined by the child rather than placed on the writing surface.

Legible writing is non-functional unless it can be reproduced in a timely manner. One of the most common concerns regarding children with handwriting dysfunction in the school setting is that they are slow and unable to complete written assignments in a specified time frame. The reasons for this are twofold. First, children with poor mechanics for writing are deterred even further when having to integrate spelling and composing into the process. Second, children with poor handwriting usually have an unstable motor set and are unable to write with automaticity and flexibility. Thus, overlearning of the legibility components is mandatory before speed can be stressed. Even then, speed may not increase for children with severe perceptual–motor difficulties. Classroom handwriting instruction at Fairley House School is consistent throughout the school and is endorsed within the remedial programme offered at the school. Letters are presented in groups of similar construction, which allows opportunities for the child with perceptual–motor difficulties to discriminate immediately between them, visually and in motor terms. The method also includes using newly learned letters in words and learning lower case letters before upper case letters. As already mentioned, children at Fairley House School are taught the cursive style of writing from the start which allows the child to deal with words as units, which also reinforces the letter patterns used in spelling. Individual letter forms are difficult to reverse and words are not easily transposed in the cursive style of writing. It is also a much faster style of writing.

Multisensory approach

By varying sensory experiences, the child's nervous system may integrate information more efficiently to produce a satisfactory motor output. Using a multisensory approach, children with perceptual–motor difficulties remain interested, challenged and enthusiastic in spite of previous failures in handwriting. All sensory systems can be tapped including the olfactory, gustatory, visual, proprioceptive, tactile and auditory senses, creating more vehicles of information arriving at the child's nervous system. When incorporating a multisensory approach, writing utensils, writing surfaces and positions for writing should all be considered in the handwriting intervention programme.

Examples of writing tools include magic markers, felt-tip pens, crayons and wipe-off crayons, pastels, weighted pens, erasable ink pens, wooden dowels and chalk. Handwriting studies on the effects of various writing tools on legibility (Lamme and Ayris, 1983) revealed that the type of writing tool did not influence legibility and the wide primary pencil did not enhance legibility any more than the adult HB pencil for beginner writers. However, the researchers noted that children's attitudes toward writing were more positive when they were able to use a felt-tip pen rather than a pencil. This suggests that a wider variety of writing tools might improve children's feelings about writing.

Writing surfaces may be in vertical or horizontal planes. Regardless of axis, writing lines are necessary to serve as direction indicators, height controllers and letter positioners. Vertical surfaces may include the chalkboard, whiteboard, laminated paper sheets and poster paper attached to the wall. An upright orientation may lessen directional confusion of letter formation for the child with perceptual–motor difficulties. On a vertical orientation, up means up and down means down, whereas on a horizontal surface, up means away from oneself and down means towards oneself. Writing on the chalkboard and laminated paper sheets also provides additional proprioceptive input, as more pressure for writing is required than the traditional paper and pencil medium.

Plastic bags filled with gel, sand trays and shaving cream are motivating horizontal writing surfaces for children. A tray filled with modelling clay can also be used as a motivating option. With a dowel stick, the child can practise letter forms in a number of different media.

Along with using a wide variety of utensils and surfaces in intervention, children's positions while writing are critical. Having total body extension in a plane parallel to the writing surface seems to allow for more internal stability of the trunk and more proprioceptive input through the upper extremities. Thus, children will benefit from standing at a vertical board while writing or lying down on a soft mat with a pillow under their chest while practising letter forms in a sand tray. Standing entails having both arms forward with slight elbow flexion, as the bases of the palms rest on the vertical surface. This posture may increase trunk control, improve proximal joint stability, promote the hand crossing the body's midline and allow a dissociation of hand movements from the forearm during writing activities. Lying prone encourages weight bearing on the forearms, which also improves proximal joint stability and enhances dissociation of the hand from the forearm while the child is engaged in forming letters. The prone position is most stressful, demanding more co-contraction through the neck and upper back musculature than either standing or sitting and tires many children quickly. Some children resist this position by lying on their side or maintaining a quadruped position.

Biomechanical approach

Sitting posture, pencil grasp and paper position are all ergonomic factors which the Occupational Therapist must attend to in the child with handwriting dysfunction. In the classroom, children spend much of their day seated at a desk which should be properly matched in size and height. Benbow (1990) recommends the child be seated at a height that allows both feet to be firmly planted on the floor, providing support for weight shifting and postural adjustments while writing. She also suggests that the desk surface be at a height 5 cm above the flexed elbow when the child is seated in the chair. This position allows the child stability and symmetry for performing written classwork.

For children with handwriting dysfunction, pencil grasp should be carefully observed. As noted earlier, an atypical grasp alone is not necessarily a precursor to poor handwriting. Functional handwriting probably has more to do with the dynamic balance of the extrinsic and intrinsic muscles and precision control than a child's prehensile pattern (Boehme, 1988).

Many prosthetic devices exist for assisting the child to develop a mature pencil grasp. Triangular pencil grips, Stetro grips, thick-barrelled pencils and Orthoplast pencil holders are all designed to encourage a tripod grasp. For the child with typically flexed fingers, an adaptive grip device or wider barrelled pencil may assist in alleviating muscle fatigue and tension when writing. Children exhibiting an incorrect grip with a static opposed thumb may benefit from a Stetro grip to correct finger positions. The focus of handwriting intervention should be placed on the balance of finger movements, making these devices transitory. If a pencil grasp is going to be modified as part of the handwriting inter-vention programme, it should occur at a young age because the longer the motor pattern is present, the more difficult it is to alter.

The position of the paper for the right-handed writer should be angled between 20° and 35° from parallel to the edge of the desk, with a slant to the left and the paper placed to the right of the midline. The mirror image is desirable for the left-handed writer. The writing utensil should be held below the line and the non-preferred hand should stabilize the writing paper. Left-handed writers may need to tilt their paper closer to 35°, allowing for better visibility of their written product.

Motivational approach

Building a positive rapport with the child is a key factor in any occupa-tional therapy intervention programme. Specific to handwriting, sharing with the child the importance of handwriting and the reasons for the intervention, such as 'We need to help your fingers catch up with your brain so you can learn how to write', may spur an initial sense of trust. Frequently, children become more motivated to exert a sincere effort when someone else invests interest in this area of their lives. The child's desire to improve handwriting should increase in an intervention programme which is filled with varied and new activities, encouragement, reinforce-ment and attainable expectations.

128   *The Occupational Therapist*

CONCLUSION

When administering a comprehensive assessment, occupational therapists must consider the underlying sensorimotor foundations of handwriting, the domains, legibility components and ergonomic factors of the child's handwriting and the interaction of the psychosocial and cognitive elements of the child's behaviour. Once these areas are determined, an integrated handwriting intervention programme can be developed by the Occupational Therapist and the educational team. Intervention programmes characterized by postural preparation of the child for writing, sequenced handwriting instruction with a variety of writing materials and media, practical biomechanical strategies for writing and encouragement and reinforcement are all successful and rewarding and create a fun environment for the child and the therapist.

References

Alton, J. and Taylor, J. (1987) *Handwriting: Theory, Research and Practice*, Croom Helm, London.
Ayres, A.J. (1966) Interrelationships among perceptual–motor functions in children. *American Journal of Occupational Therapy*, **20**, 288–92.
Ayres, A.J. (1969) Deficits in sensory integration in educationally handicapped children. *Journal of Learning Disabilities*, **2**, 160–8.
Ayres, A.J. (1985) Developmental dyspraxia and adult onset dyspraxia. A lecture prepared for Sensory Integration International by A. Jean Ayres PhD.
Beery, K.E. (1982) *Administration, Scoring and Teaching Manual for the Developmental Test of Visual–Motor Integration*, Modern Curriculum Press, Cleveland, Ohio.
Benbow, M. (1990) *Loops and Other Groups*, Therapy Skill Builders, Tucson, Arizona.
Bergman, K.E. and McLaughlin, T.F. (1988) Remediating handwriting difficulties with learning disabled students: a review. *British Columbia Journal of Special Education*, **12**(2), 101–20.
Boehme, R. (1988) *Improving Upper Body Control*, Therapy Skill Builders, Tucson, Arizona.
Carrow-Woolfolk, E. (1981) *Carrow Auditory–Visual Abilities Test Manual*, Teaching Resources Corporation, New York.
Exner, C.E. (1989) Development of hand functions. In *Occupational Therapy for Children* (eds P.N. Pratt and A.S. Allen), C.V. Mosby, St. Louis, pp. 235–59.
Exner, C.E. (1992) In-hand manipulation skills. In *Development of Hand Skills in the Child* (eds J. Case-Smith and C. Pehoski), American Occupational Therapy Association, Rockville.
Gubbay, S.S. (1978) The management of developmental dyspraxia. *Developmental Medicine and Child Neurology*, **20**, 643–6.
Henderson, S.E. and Sugden, D.A. (1992) *Movement Assessment Battery for*

Children Manual, The Psychological Corporation/Harcourt Brace Jovanovich, New York.

Jordan, B.T. (1980) *Jordan Left–Right Reversal Test Manual*. Novato, California, Academic Therapy Publications.

Lamme, L.L. and Ayris, B.M. (1983) Is the handwriting of beginning writers influenced by writing tools? *Journal of Research and Development in Education*, **17**(1), 33–8.

McGourty, L.K., Foto, M., Marvin, J.K. *et al.* (1989) *Uniform Terminology for Occupational Therapy*, 2nd edn, American Occupational Therapy Association, Rockville.

Peck, M., Askov, E.N. and Fairchild, S.H. (1980) Another decade of research in handwriting: progress and prospect in the 1970s. *Journal of Educational Research*, **73**(5), 283–98.

Wechsler, D. (1976) *Wechsler Intelligence Scale for Children – Revised*. Windsor: NFER.

Further reading

Amundson, S.J.C. (1992) Handwriting: evaluation and intervention in school settings. In *Development of Hand Skills in the Child* (eds J. Case-Smith and C. Petroski), American Occupational Therapy Association, Rockville.

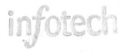

5 The Orthoptist

Ann Wilson

Ann Wilson is an Orthoptist with considerable experience and skill on whose services the school calls at regular intervals for advice on visual anomalies. Her diagnostic inputs are immensely valuable to parents and specialist staff alike. Her work frequently allows a child to be visually very much better prepared for the considerable undertaking that is involved in dealing with specific learning disabilities.

P.G.

Introduction

Essentially, the work of an Orthoptist concerns itself with the functioning of the visual system. At Fairley House, this involves the anomalies that may arise in the particular group of children who have specific learning difficulties.

We need to look not only at visual acuity, or in other words the actual quality of sight, but also at the considerable variety of ocular malfunctions which can occur and hinder visual processing, making the life of the child very much more difficult. However, we must also give thought to the child's capacity to process the information once it has been received by the visual system.

The work of the Orthoptist will bring her into contact with patients of a variety of ages from the preschool years through to adulthood. The three examples which will be discussed in this chapter are in no way exclusive; neither do they address all the difficulties that may well arise in an assessment. Their problems and a number of other ocular conditions which do not appear in these examples will be discussed at the end of each section, as well as an explanation of the technical terms used. Nevertheless, these three children were quite typical and not only demonstrate the teamwork approach but also show quite clearly the tremendous advantage of early diagnosis, as in all three cases the eventual outcome was entirely satisfactory.

Susan

I had known Susan since she was 1 year old. She presented with a congenital right convergent squint with right amblyopia (right lazy eye due to the squint). She was found to be considerably hypermetropic with some astigmatism (see later text) and glasses were prescribed. She was then successfully treated, first by occlusion (patching) to equalize her vision and then by surgery to correct the position of her eyes.

At the age of 4½ she was ready for school. She still wore glasses, but her vision in both eyes was normal and equal. Memories of surgery and patching were almost forgotten. She was a particularly bright and articulate little girl, who always cooperated well when being tested. She started school enthusiastically, with high parental expectations.

Her enthusiasm for school, however, soon disappeared and she became almost school phobic. She failed to recognize her alphabet visually – although she could sing it well! – and her pencil control and drawings were below par. It came to the stage when she would refuse even to try to write or copy.

She came for a routine eye examination at 5½ years of age and I asked about her school progress. My enquiry unleashed a torrent of parental concern. I was able to explain to her mother and father, and subsequently to her most cooperative teacher, that a right-handed child with a right-sided squint (i.e. left eye dominant) is likely to have poor visual perception, poor visual memory and visuo-motor integration and poor hand control, especially if the squint is associated with hypermetropia and/or astigmatism. The teacher had not even realized that Susan had squinted.

The method of teaching Susan was changed from a system based on 'look and say' to a more structured phonics-based, yet multisensory approach. Her auditory skills were excellent. 'Big' letter patterns were introduced, allowing the child, for example, to use a relaxed whole arm on a blackboard or even a window. Games and activities to encourage her hand–eye coordination and visual perception were played at school and at home. Number concepts were introduced using concrete, everyday objects and this again was reinforced at home. She was also helped to develop a compensatory technique for copying both at near and far distances.

Susan herself was made aware of just why she had had difficulty – her parents and teachers worked in tandem – and at her last routine eye test she presented as a happy little girl, enjoying her school and making excellent progress.

Careful observation and assessment of Susan revealed two core issues.

- Congenital right convergent squint with right amblyopia (right lazy eye due to the squint), subsequently treated by occlusion (Fig. 5.1) and surgery.
- Hypermetropia with some astigmatism (see later text).

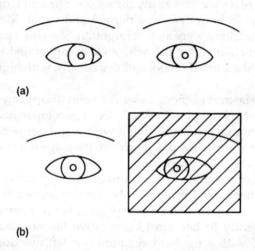

Fig. 5.1 (a) Right convergent squint; (b) right eye forced into action by occlusion of the left eye.

Ocular motor balance

Normally the two eyes are held straight by the eye muscles and are well balanced. There is usually a slight underlying tendency to deviate very marginally from the absolutely straight (orthophoric) position, but this is held in check by the innate desire of the brain to maintain binocular, single vision.

If this balance and control is lost a squint (**strabismus**) will result. This can be horizontal, with the eye turning inwards (**esotropia**, a convergent squint) or outwards (**exotropia**, a divergent squint). Alternatively, the deviation can be vertical hypertropia or a combination of horizontal and vertical elements. The squint can be marked and readily observable or so small as to be hardly apparent to the casual observer.

At the outset of a squint, double vision (**diplopia**) occurs but this, in childhood, is quickly suppressed. If the same eye is always suppressed then this eye is very likely to become 'lazy' (**amblyopic**) – once again apparent as part of Susan's diagnosis. Due to early and regular screening, diagnosis of squint is now made soon after onset and early treatment is encouraged. However, it is important that teachers are made aware of the earlier condition and its treatment, as children with an early squint are often clumsy, with poor hand–eye coordination. In turn, this causes difficulty with visuo-spatial concepts. Visual memory may be poor and the child struggles to recognize the shape of a word, although he may be aware that he has seen it many times before. Copying difficulties will often present as a presumed visual problem in an eye clinic.

If there is no actual squint but the ocular imbalance is significant and control difficult, then there may also be consequent visual problems. Under conditions of stress binocular vision may be lost, resulting in either double vision or loss of stereoscopic vision due to the suppression of one eye. It is important that both the clumsiness and the eye condition are perceived as lying within a single syndrome in these circumstances, as they may well both be connected to the child's literacy difficulties. So often this is not fully realized and each is treated as a separate entity.

Treatment of the ocular muscle imbalance does not, unfortunately, immediately cure the visuo-spatial difficulties since these are long-standing, but understanding the problem is vital when planning the child's remedial programme. One would anticipate improvement once comfortable binocular vision has been properly established.

Hypermetropia

In this condition the dioptric mechanism of the eye is too weak – the eye is relatively too short and parallel rays of light are not brought to a focus on the retina without an effort of accommodation (focusing). Small children normally have a degree of physiological hypermetropia which reduces with growth. By 6–7 years of age children should have normal refraction. Children have ample accommodation available to them, so that hypermetropia alone can be overcome by an effort of accommodation and distance vision will usually appear normal. However, as accommodation and convergence are linked, the balance between the two eyes can be upset, producing discomfort, headaches and, in some cases, a convergent squint when attempting to read.

Especially in children with specific learning difficulties, any significant degree of hypermetropia should be corrected even though vision itself may appear unimpaired. There is evidence that perception time is quicker when refraction is corrected, even though the uncorrected visual acuity may appear to be the same. This condition is frequently overlooked at routine school eye checks where only visual acuity for distance is recorded.

Glasses should be worn for all close work at home and at school.

Myopia

Poor distance vision may be due to myopia, or short sight. The refracting media of the eye are relatively too powerful – the eye is too long and a blurred image of a distant object is formed on the retina.

Myopia can occur with growth, so that an eye that appears to see perfectly normally at six years of age may have become significantly myopic at seven and distance vision will have dropped quite dramatically.

A surprisingly small degree of myopia causes a very significant drop in distance vision. For near work, however, the moderate myope should have perfect vision without making any accommodative effort. It is hardly surprising, therefore, that many myopes prefer to read without glasses but, nevertheless, in the classroom, where focus is rapidly changing from one distance to another, glasses should be worn.

A child who is constantly screwing up his eyes to see the board should always be suspected of being myopic. The condition varies in its age of onset and progression, but while growth is occurring refraction should be very regular, especially if there is a family history of myopia.

Astigmatism

In the astigmatic, the eye is oval instead of being spherical. It can be associated with varying degrees of hypermetropia or myopia or, indeed, a combination of the two (mixed astigmatism).

If the degree of astigmatism is large then visual acuity will be reduced considerably. With only a slight degree of astigmatism, however, vision may appear acceptable, but in some individuals it will bring with it headaches and visual discomfort or an abnormal head posture due to an unsuccessful attempt to obtain clear vision. Correction with cylindrical lenses should produce clear, normal vision without symptoms.

Anisometropia

In this instance there is a difference between the refraction of the two eyes and as the nervous impulse to both eyes has to be identical, one eye has to be used more than the other. In some cases, if not treated, the disadvantaged eye will become lazy or amblyopic and require treatment in order to restore vision. Where there is an associated reading difficulty, all significant cases of anisometropia should be corrected with glasses, especially if the weaker eye is on the side of the preferred hand, since this may prevent effective lateralization. Sometimes, one eye is preferred for distance and the other for near work until the refractive condition is corrected.

Extraocular movements

The eyes are moved by six muscles, four rectus (straight) muscles and two oblique muscles to each eye. The eyes should move equally and smoothly together in all positions of the gaze to maintain comfortable, binocular, single vision in all directions.

Sometimes, one or more of these muscles can be damaged, often from birth. Either a squint will develop or, at times, a compensatory head position will be sought in order to maintain binocular vision. The head is turned or tilted so that the offending muscle does not have to be used. This condition has clear implications as to where the child should be positioned physically in class. With blackboard work or even sharing a book with a neighbour, the teacher must be careful that the child is placed so that visual learning is from the direction of the unaffected eye muscles. Once again, it is important to stress the tremendous importance of a multidisciplinary approach in the diagnosis and management of this difficulty and of the regular need for liaison between classteachers, parents and all other professionals.

These children are, again, often clumsy with poor visual–motor skills and poor visual short-term sequential memory (handwriting and copying difficulties).

Accommodation

This is the ability of the eye to increase the dioptric power of its lens in order to bring the image of a near object into focus. There is a normal range for each age and if the amplitude is reduced, hypermetropia should be suspected in the first instance and the child should have a careful refraction test using cycloplegic drops. These temporarily dilate the pupil and prevent accommodation so that an accurate and purely objective measurement of refraction can be made.

Eric

Eric was 9 years old when I first met him. He was failing badly at school where his classteacher thought he was stupid. There was a family history of early reading problems, poor spelling and also Eric himself had been born three months prematurely with a very low birth weight.

His development, however, had been good. He was an early talker and presented as a well-grown, normal little boy. He was very able verbally, but extremely stressed and unhappy about his total lack of progress at school which was causing considerable concern. He too thought he was stupid.

Closer questioning revealed that Eric was very clumsy, both in fine and gross motor movements. He was left-handed with poor pencil control and his 'writing' was illegible. He had never been referred for any assessment, since, in those very early years following his premature birth, speech and language development had been excellent and he had demonstrated a wide vocabulary.

There was a history of a late start in Eric's reading. He had been slow to recognize his letters and sight words had proved impossible. He just did not recognize them. However, around six years there had been a sudden and dramatic improvement as he learned a phonic approach. At nine he was an avid reader, but testing revealed that his reading was inaccurate and that he scanned badly, using context cues to guess difficult words.

Eric's spelling was appalling – though it followed the phonic rules at a basic level – his 'writing' was illegible and number concepts were nil. His sense of body image was poor and he would get lost walking from one classroom to another. He was not able to copy from the board. Hence, his sight was questioned.

His vision was, in fact, normal. He had normal eye balance and binocular function and convergence, but his following (tracking) movements were unsteady and jerky and his scanning poor. He was almost entirely ambilateral, but chose to write with his left hand. His balance and coordination generally were noted as weak.

Eric was referred to the Occupational Therapist, who confirmed his motor difficulties. Remedial help was started at school and at home, with his mother and remedial teacher working in tandem. His coordination and pencil control improved and he learned a technique for copying correctly. Spelling improved slowly and steadily, but it was his maths which caused the greatest heartache, especially over concepts such as fractions, area and the decimal system. With help his anxiety gradually decreased and slowly he began to enjoy school. It is not widely understood that severe maths difficulties can be very much a part of the broad dyslexic syndrome.

When Eric was assessed by the Educational Psychologist his performance scale IQ was found to be more than 40 points lower than his verbal skills, but with help he has achieved academic success. His headmistress spoke of him recently as being one of her most gifted children. His future looks good. He is a happy teenager.

The issues that arise from our observations of Eric concern:

- preliminary eye testing, which in his case produced normal vision, eye muscle balance, binocular function and good binocular convergence;
- scanning – found to be poor;
- laterality – uncertain;
- balance and coordination difficulties – requiring referral to an Occupational Therapist.

Binocular function

This is the ability to use the two eyes as a pair to produce a single image. It must be carefully tested and should be well developed. Exercises may be advised in some cases, where the eyes do not work together as they should.

BINOCULAR CONVERGENCE

It is important that all children with a reading difficulty have a normal range of smooth, well-controlled binocular convergence. This is the ability to keep the eyes directed steadily at the object of fixation as it approaches the nose. Again, exercises may be advised for some children. Poor convergence can cause a reading problem in itself.

Assessment of visual acuity

Children are normally referred because a visual problem of some kind has been detected by either the parents or teachers. It may even be simply to exclude possible visual anomalies, as part of a full and detailed assessment, as would be the case in Fairley House.

Suspicions may arise in class where a child seems to have exaggerated difficulty with far-point copying, i.e. from the board, or struggles to keep his place in a line of print. He may seem to peer at a distant target and at the end of a school day may be much given to eye rubbing and fatigue. The child may also hold his head at a strange angle or complain that words look blurred or jumbled.

In the case of the Orthoptist, the decision needs to be made as to whether these problems are caused by a visual dysfunction or by a difficulty of visual processing (see also Chapters 2 and 4). However, it must be remembered that, at times, the two can be thoroughly interrelated. It is quite apparent that a fully detailed diagnostic picture will seldom be available without the individual input of several professionals representing interrelated disciplines.

Eye testing for visual acuity should be managed very carefully and thoroughly. It is important to check both eyes together in the first instance and then with each individual eye separately for near and distance vision. The chart that the child is reading should be changed, as even dyslexic children sometimes manage to memorize a line of letters and this can so easily lead to misdiagnosis. Equally, each eye in its turn should be carefully occluded to avoid peeping.

It sometimes emerges that when each eye is used on its own, acuity seems unimpaired, but there is a difficulty in using the eyes together due, most frequently, to a muscle imbalance between the two eyes or to unequal refractive error. It is important to note any abnormal head posture and/or a tendency to screw up one or both eyes. We occasionally observe 'wobbling' eyes in a child (**nystagmus**). Vision may be good when both eyes are used together, but their effectiveness is reduced markedly when either eye is occluded.

Some children may not know the letter sounds or the written letter symbols associated with them but this problem can be overcome either by using a picture chart or, preferably, a matching letter chart. Children of average ability can match well enough to test at just over two years of age, so that an early accurate, subjective assessment of vision can be obtained. However, care must be taken with any shape which could be reversed or one which could easily be confused by a child with poor visuo-perceptual skills. It is up to the Orthoptist to decide whether errors are due to poor visual discrimination or poor visual acuity.

Especially with children with specific learning disabilities, it is vital to check whether a child actually needs to have each letter pointed out separately in turn. So many of these children can see better than adequately, but are quite unable to scan along a line without losing their place.

A child may come to an eye clinic saying that he cannot see the board and that his eyes tire very quickly when attempting to read. At times, poor visual acuity is recorded and the child is subsequently referred to an Ophthalmologist for an objective refraction, discussed earlier in the chapter. At this test eye drops will be used to prevent subjective focusing by the child. Usually a refractive error is found and glasses are prescribed accordingly.

However, occasionally, no abnormality whatever is found and the child's eyes appear perfectly healthy and no refractive error is recorded. The symptoms then usually prove to be 'hysterical' in origin, caused by stress, often associated with poor reading and spelling. 'If I cannot see, I cannot be expected to read, so no one will get cross with me.' This response is seldom made at a conscious level but lurks beneath the surface within the subconscious. The symptom of poor vision in this case is quite literally a 'cry for help' and it is so very important that the child is not dismissed with a simplistic label – 'no problem'.

Poor vision in itself is unlikely to cause a reading problem. There are many partially sighted children who achieve very high standards in their literacy skills, but it is vital that a child with a learning problem has as good vision as possible. It is also important that any difference in vision between the two eyes is corrected, since it may be a contributing factor in a lack of proper lateralization.

Scanning

In Eric's case, his scanning was poor and his following movements were unsteady. He had also failed to establish a reference eye at this point in his development.

REFERENCE EYE

The reference eye is not the same as the dominant or 'telescopic' eye, where we are examining a monocular task, when one eye is chosen in preference to the other. This is the dominant eye; only one eye is being used.

However, when a child is reading, the eyes should assume a convergent position. The visual axes are, therefore, no longer parallel, each having a separate visual direction. The brain receives two sets of information: visual information, which is received from both retinae and which is then sent to both occipital cortices in the brain, and proprioceptive information, which informs visual direction. As this direction is different in the two eyes, one must consistently take the lead in order that the eyes can scan smoothly along a line of print, reading the words and the letters in the correct orientation. The eye that takes this lead is called the reference eye. Once this has been clearly established it provides reliable and consistent ocular-motor/retinal information to the brain; in other words, it correlates what the eyes are seeing with where it is in space (so 'was' will not be read as 'saw').

THE DUNLOP TEST

This test is used to diagnose whether or not a reference eye has been established. It was first used by Patricia Dunlop in Australia, in 1970. Fig. 5.2 demonstrates the use of a synotophore, or adapted stereoscope, with subjective–objective control arms. This is the instrument used to conduct the Dunlop Test. Two slides are inserted, one for each eye, and, using the arms, the patient joins them so that he sees a single image but with two controls – one from each eye. The tubes are then moved slowly and equally outwards, so that fusion of the two slides cannot be maintained. Just before fusion breaks there should be an illusion that one or other of the controls moves and the other one stays still. (This is called the 'autokinetic effect' and was first described by Ogle in 1954.)

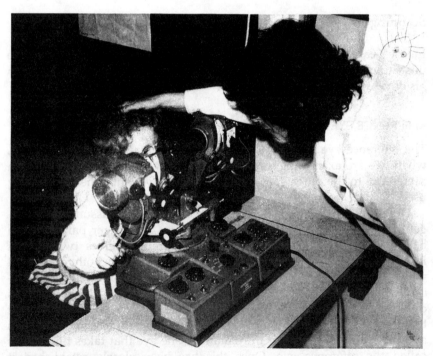

Fig. 5.2 The synotophore.

The test should be repeated ten times. If a reference eye has been established it will always be the control of the same eye which is seen to stay still. A nine out of ten response in favour of one eye means that this can be considered to be the established (fixed) reference eye.

It is claimed that unstable responses to the Dunlop Test indicate that a child has failed to make reliable ocular-motor/retinal association.

Stein and Fowler (1985) discovered that at 6 years of age 60% of the normal population showed a fixed reference eye and after this there is a 10% increase each year. In principle one would expect a reference eye to be established by the time the normal child is expected to read. Clearly this moment in the child's development will vary in each individual, depending on ability among other factors.

There are one or two difficulties that need to be addressed in the case of reference eye work. First and foremost, dyslexic children are often feeling stressed and anxious already and further investigation does not help their anxiety levels. Hence, they will often be very keen to please and this will distort responses. Furthermore, significant numbers of children with specific learning disabilities also experience an attention deficit and this makes concentration on this comparatively complex task almost beyond them.

However, with care, sensitivity and patience it is usually possible to help these children achieve a satisfactory response. It is also fair to say that a percentage of children and adults never establish a reference eye and yet appear to read adequately. However, on closer examination it would appear that although the vast majority of these subjects have very efficient phoneme–grapheme analysis they depend very heavily on context cues. Experimentally, when they are asked to read nonsense words or words without any context, especially if these are polysyllabic, they experience far more difficulty than one would generally expect because they are unable to scan adequately.

TREATMENT TO ESTABLISH A REFERENCE EYE

If there is unfixed reference, occlusion should be worn whilst scanning exercises are carried out. The scanning card should be prepared by the teacher and produced at the precise level to suit the particular needs of the child.

Opinions differ as to how much occlusion should be worn but we feel that this should be for short, regular periods each day while the child is reading a non-context scanning card – non-context because this prevents anticipation or guessing of words and forces the child to read from left to right. Absolute accuracy is essential. The cards will need to be changed very often as progress is made, to prevent memorization. Occlusion should never be carried out without professional advice.

The following are one-line examples taken from phonic scan sheets made specifically, at the correct level, for individual children (real or nonsense words and syllables can be used):

Example 1 – at up et me no ot en og go
Example 2 – cat pin dog pat nip tin pit dug
Example 3 – sindin banden bigding setmat cotpindog
Example 4 – at ate ip ot ipe ote um on ute ut
Example 5 – oot out at oat on oin oy oon
Example 6 – oping iling apping illing opping iming
Example 7 – carfilling bountiful pointingless winchinning

Cursive letter patterns and other tracking exercises can also be carried out whilst the occlusion is worn.

By the time the child has finished a series of exercises of this kind he should find it possible to scan much more easily and evenly from left to right, without letter or word reversals/transposals.

Colour coding can also prove very effective, both for emphasizing the appropriate vowels and also separating the syllables. It is important, however, to ensure that the child is not colour blind; 8% of boys show some difficulty with colour vision. A colour vision test should always be included in the battery of tests.

As the exercise becomes more sophisticated, so increasingly similar words can be used to stimulate visual discrimination and the child should be encouraged to chunk the sounds, rather than pronounce each letter sound individually. Research is currently being carried out using computer-based infra-red tracking equipment, so that all eye movements can be recorded and the findings can be analysed. This will assist considerably in the diagnosis and treatment of tracking difficulties. There is also some evidence that coloured lenses and coloured overlays also help a child to stabilize the print and reduce scanning and tracking difficulties. Much has been written about the condition known as 'scotopic sensitivity syndrome'. This is said to be a defect causing loss of sensitivity to a particular part of the retina. Specially tinted lenses may help to alleviate the problem. The Irlin Institute was possibly the first to introduce the concept and several centres are now involved in detailed research.

It would seem sensible to try the selection of coloured acetate overlays in the initial stages, to assess the degree to which the child responds, before embarking on lengthy assessment and prescription of coloured lenses. Clearly an assessment of effectiveness in this situation is purely subjective and relies very much on the response and involvement of the child. A significant number of normal children and, indeed, adults find a coloured overlay extremely helpful.

If the chosen overlay produces a convincing improvement then glasses can be made up in the appropriate colour.

Laterality

Eric was ambilateral in that he appeared able to use both sides of his body with equal effect, but chose to write with his left hand.

The laterality should be observed and assessed by the Orthoptist, the Psychologist or the Occupational Therapist, all of whom are trained to observe and record in some detail the preferred hand, eye, foot and ear.

A significant number of children with specific learning disabilities are, in fact, crosslateral. For example, a youngster may be right-handed but have a dominant left eye and while this may present no particular learning problem, a significant number of these children have a history of slight developmental delay in literacy skills. There is also a marked tendency to confuse concepts like sequence and direction. The greatest problem, however, arises when a child is unsure of which hand or eye to use. It is surprising how often one observes a 'unicorn response' in that the child places the tube, through which he should be looking with his chosen eye, in the middle of the forehead! Equally, the child may be completely uncertain and uncommitted as to which eye to choose. It is also of considerable significance if a child chooses to hold his head at a great angle in order to look through the tube or has to hold the other eye shut in order to look through the dominant eye.

The clumsy child, whose laterality is not established or who is cross-lateral, frequently demonstrates visuo-spatial difficulties and problems of visuo-motor integration and may also exhibit poor visual memory.

Balance and coordination are looked at in detail by the Occupational Therapist, but are also observed by the Orthoptist as the child moves around the office, climbs on and off the examination chair or picks up and uses the objects which form part of the test. In most circumstances children will be asked to draw, partly to help them relax and partly to give the Orthoptist an opportunity to observe their fine motor skills and the way in which they hold their pencil.

Jane
Jane was 6½ when I first met her. She thought herself stupid and was distressed by school. She was a healthy child with a history of normal development. Her only medical problems had been tonsillectomy/adenoidectomy at 4½ years of age, following persistent tonsillitis.

On closer questioning, however, several other important factors emerged. She had been a very early talker with a wide vocabulary, but her early speech was only intelligible to her family. By nearly school age she was well understood, so no intervention had been advised. Although not clumsy in the accepted sense (she was very neat and precise and could make excellent models and drawings), she often 'fell over her own feet' and refused to join her friends in ballet class because she was 'always on the wrong foot'. She had been ambidextrous until about 4 years of age, finally deciding to be right-handed. She had been a messy eater as a toddler, but again by school age her hand control was good. She often 'lost her way' and would tend to panic if there was no one to follow.

School was becoming more and more difficult. She was able to recognize some of her letters, but muddled b/d/p/q; m/w; n/u/h and would often start writing from the right-hand side of the page. Number symbols were impossible because 19 might be produced as 91, 61 or even 16. Again, she never knew where to start. Her knowledge of sight words was almost non-existent and she seemed to be unable to copy from the board.

Eye examination revealed normal vision, binocular function and normal eye movements, but with the characteristic 'mid-line jump'. She was right-handed superficially, but really ambidextrous with no established reference. She scanned poorly and had a very poor visual sequential memory and poor directional skills.

Remedial help was started, including some occlusion, with great success but it was a long time before her self-image improved and she was able to believe that she was as intelligent as her friends – if not more so.

Issues arising from Jane's case include:

- normal vision and binocular function and eye movements, but characteristic mid-line jump;
- no established reference;
- poor scanning;
- very poor visual sequential memory;
- poor directional skills.

Mid-line jump

In the case of mixed or uncertain laterality there is often an inability to follow a fixation target across the mid-line of the body if the head is kept still. This is said to be due to difficulty in passing all the relevant information from one hemisphere of the brain to the other.

For a subject whose neurology is already rather different from that of a normally learning child, this mid-line difficulty may well make scanning either a line of print or tasks such as catching a ball surprisingly difficult.

Reference eye

We have discussed the significance of an unestablished reference eye at some length in Eric's case and Jane, once again, experienced very similar difficulties. Indeed, the failure to establish a reference eye features remarkably often in the profile of children with specific learning difficulties.

Poor scanning

Here again the patterns are not dissimilar, as is so often the case, but as Jane was only 6½, age was even more in her favour.

Visual sequential memory and directional skills

In essence, this implies the ability to remember spatial orientation without verbal or logical clues. In other words there is no apparent sense or theme underlying the symbols that must be retained. It is simply a matter of recalling visually in which order they will fall.

This will be tested in great detail by the Occupational Therapist and Psychologist and the topic is dealt with in Chapters 2 and 4.

Conclusion

By now it will be quite apparent that any investigation of visual phenomena is a much more complex issue than simply ascertaining whether an individual can see well with both eyes. It is also clear that a wide variety of possible visual anomalies need to be investigated and the significance, possible treatment and management discussed with teachers and other specialist staff concerned so that an appropriate remedial programme can be planned to produce maximum effect.

It is obviously of crucial importance that all those working with children with specific learning disabilities are well aware of exactly what difficulties each child is experiencing in all modalities and the effect these will have on learning and, more extensively, on performance in class as a whole and also on behaviour and attitude at home.

146   *The Orthoptist*

Further reading

Dunlop, D.B. and Dunlop, P. (1972) The binocular basis of dyslexic confusion. *Australian Orthoptic Journal*, 12, 16–20.

Dunlop, D.B., Dunlop, P. and Fenelon, B. (1973) Vision – laterality analysis in children with reading disability: the results of new techniques of examination. *Cortex*, 9, 227–36.

Ogle, K. (1962) Optical space sense, in H. Davson (ed.) *The Eye*, Volume 4, Norton, New York.

Stein, J.F. and Fowler, M.S. (1985) The effect of monocular occlusion on visuomotor perception and reading in dyslexic children. *Lancet*, 13, 69–72.

6 The Paediatrician

Dr Sam Tucker

Dr Tucker is a Consultant Paediatrician of considerable experience. He is a Consultant to the school which he visits from time to time, offering valuable support and advice, largely based on classroom observation and case conferences with the relevant staff. At times, the queries raised will lead to clinical referral to Dr Tucker, appropriate paediatric investigation and advice to both parents and the school. He has also been a valuable guide to possible avenues of research in the future into the understanding and management of specific learning disabilities.

P.G.

Aetiology of dyslexia

There are basically two main causes of dyslexia.

1. GENETIC

It is now a general finding that a family history of dyslexia is present in over 50% of the families studied (Hallgren, 1987). What appears to have been inherited is not a reading disability per se, but aspects of phonological processing (Candor *et al.*, 1994).

Genetic evidence of linkage on chromosome 15 and for markers on chromosome 1 has been reported in dyslexic families and recently linkage on chromosome 6. Further work on this is in progress.

Genetic linkage occurs when two gene loci are physically close together on the chromosome. A diseased or defective gene will be linked to a particular type within a given affected family, but will not necessarily be associated with the same antigens in unaffected related people. Specific typing can be used to predict disease or defects by establishing the linked type within a given family. 'Linkage' is the term describing genes or DNA sequences situated close together on the same chromosome that tend to segregate together.

'Marker' is the general term used for biochemical or DNA poly-morphism (the genetic characteristic with more than one common form in the population), occurring close to a gene and used in gene tracking.

2. NEUROLOGICAL

Many children, having developed normal spoken language, often without intellectual impairment, may experience aphasia (loss of under-standing of words) as a result of brain injury or lesion, but this is not true of the vast majority of dyslexics.

There is no adequate evidence in the literature to incriminate other conditions such as prematurity, babies who are small for gestational age, obstetric difficulties or jaundice.

HEMISPHERIC CONTROL IN DYSLEXIA

Dyslexia is thought to be due to deviations from the normal hemispheric development in the brain of the learning to read process (Bakker, 1987). Initial reading is primarily dependent on right hemispheric processing. This produces slow, rather analytic reading as opposed to advanced, fluent reading which is mediated by the left hemisphere. This primary control of reading switches from right to left hemisphere at some point during the normal development of the learning to read process, usually after one or two years of reading experience. If children fail to make the shift, they go on relying on the right hemisphere strategies associated with slow reading. Some children may even use left hemisphere strate-gies from the start of learning to read, thereby skipping the phase of initial reading which would have required right hemisphere control.

Nootropic drugs (drugs acting on the central nervous system), e.g. Piracetam (Conners, 1987), have been reported to facilitate speed of reading in this group, where the right hemisphere requires stimulation to encourage the switch to the left. Further research is now continuing into the cognitive effects of this medication in some types of dyslexics. Piracetam seems to work by facilitating information processing for linguistic stimuli and these changes can be reflected in electro-physiological measurement.

Physical evaluation

While the routine physical and neurological examination is often normal, examination of indices of central nervous system function such as laterality, mirror phenomena, choreiform movements and performance on a variety of fine and gross motor tasks is often helpful. Although each of these indicators or neuromaturational signs is considered to be minor in nature and often occurs in normal children, they are not usually related to any structural nervous system abnormality. Tests relying solely on gross motor ability, handedness, dominance and choreiform syndromes would be ineffective in identifying affected children from normals.

In addition to the child's history, physical and neurological examination, psychometric testing is frequently helpful in the evaluation of the child. This will enable a better understanding of any other learning problems such as attention deficits. If the paediatrician is to become an effective and responsible advocate for children with learning problems, he must become adept at interpreting these tools.

Specialized tests, such as electroencephalography (EEG) and computed tomography (CT), have not provided us with evidence of brain dysfunction and other investigative measures (haematological indices, biochemical parameters, endocrine studies) have not proved clinically useful.

Children with specific learning difficulties may present to the paediatrician with a variety of psychosomatic symptoms such as headaches, abdominal pain and visual difficulties. A detailed family history may be adequate to uncover and help diagnose dyslexia or other learning difficulties. There is no sense in waiting to see how the child develops, because any delay in starting to read can subsequently develop into a significant learning disorder.

Hearing impairment of any severity must always be considered and excluded by specialized testing. Sensorineural deafness will inevitably have a serious effect on the reception of auditory information and the earlier the diagnosis is confirmed and a rehabilitative programme put into place, the sooner will the infant or child learn to speak as do other children.

The ability of secretory or serous otitis media (glue ear) to delay or inhibit language development is more controversial. Over 30% of children under five will have at least one attack and a considerable number will experience many more. If the fluid in the middle ear persists for lengthy periods and treatment has not been very effective, speech and language impairment may occur if there is a persistent hearing loss. This must be identified quickly and remedied. The association between serous otitis media and permanent hearing loss is by no means proven and studies are continuing in this field.

Seizures are always a possible cause of intellectual deterioration and with the correct treatment, the learning problem often disappears. Petit mal attacks are just such an example; because of the frequent momentary losses of consciousness, they need to be differentiated from daydreaming. Progressive neurological disorders must be recognized so that treatment can be initiated if available. Lead poisoning should be considered in the younger child and alcoholism or other drug abuse may contribute to the problem in the older child.

Physical evidence suggestive of child abuse requires intervention and intensive follow-up. Severe depression is not that uncommon in childhood but does need detection and medical management. The acute or subacute onset of a learning problem should alert one to the possibility of infectious, toxic or traumatic processes and focal neurological signs may be detectable. Many patterns of abnormal behaviour, especially in learning disorders, can cause diagnostic confusion. Asperger's syndrome and infantile autism, for example, are in many ways similar and there is much discussion as to whether they are varieties of the same underlying abnormality or two separate entities.

Attention deficits in dyslexia

Many dyslexic children have problems associated with concentration in the school environment and their inability to maintain attention will adversely influence reading and writing competence. Motor control may also be compromised and may interfere with handwriting and other skills.

Attention deficit disorder (ADD) (Barkley, 1990) is a developmental disorder of behavioural inhibition. There is a significant developmental delay in age-appropriate control of behaviour resulting in deficits in sustained attention, impulse control, rule-governed behaviour and the regulation of activity level as demanded by various situations. This disorder is significantly pervasive, has an onset in early childhood, is chronic throughout development and is not due to mental retardation or brain damage. ADD is now considered to be a physiologically-based disorder as opposed to deliberate misbehaviour, though 'misbehaviours' may often become a significant part of the problem.

There are basically two main types of ADD – with hyperactivity and impulsivity (ADHD) and inattention (ADD). Children with ADHD have great difficulty in focusing and sustaining their attention, as well as regulating their behaviour. They are impulsive and disinhibited, restless and disruptive with mood problems.

Case study
Alexander had been difficult since birth and his mother commented that his constant movements and kicking in the womb had caused her much discomfort before delivery. As a baby, he was difficult to feed and developed infantile colic very early. He did not need much sleep, unlike his mother. He cried excessively and was very demanding of his mother's time. He was a real handful. During the 'terrible twos' period, comforted and reassured by

doctors that this was normal behaviour for his age, his mother still felt unhappy as his communication level was poor and his speech and language were rather immature. The parents were given endless suggestions on how to cope both by professionals and well-meaning friends but nothing seemed to improve things. At the end of each day his mother was completely exhausted.

On occasions he was a delight to be with and his mother could cope with the odd little problem but on most days, his behaviour was unacceptable and unmanageable. At times he could not complete the simplest of tasks where previously he had succeeded without much difficulty. Despite love and attention, Alexander never seemed to be satisfied and his demands were always increasing. He became more frustrated and bored. Mood swings were appearing more often and he threw temper tantrums whenever he was asked to carry out even simple tasks. His ability to sense danger was minimal and he would do things which were entirely inappropriate. He would act first, usually impulsively, and then wonder about the sense of the action, often far too late. Explanations resulted in further wild activities and he often ran amok in the supermarket, causing havoc and considerable embarrassment.

Alexander could not maintain an attention span for any significant period of time and could not always recall what had just been asked of him. At kindergarten and later at school, Alexander was more aggressive than other children and because of this antisocial behaviour, became very unpopular. His parents were at their wits' end and their marriage was threatened.

In the classroom Alexander was disruptive and distractible and concentration was not possible for more than a very few minutes. He was always in trouble with teachers and fellow students. Everyone felt he had the potential and on some days he achieved his best work. This, however, was the exception rather than the rule. He impressed while using the computer. His organizational ability was very poor. His self-esteem deteriorated and he fell behind in his schoolwork. He had already changed schools twice. His whole future was now at risk.

Attention deficit disorder (ADD) children, unlike Alexander, have few problems controlling their behaviour and are not usually hyperactive. In fact, they usually go unnoticed in a classroom as they create no conflict, no difficulty and are usually the 'daydreamers'. Their failure to achieve good academic levels results from poor sustained attention and difficulty in focusing on a given task.

Case study

Samantha was a shy, quiet, introverted girl who was always co-operative and helpful, but was noted as a 'dreamer'. To attract and maintain her attention was a problem and instructions would have to be repeated many times before she was able to perform the task requested. She was often a loner and could play on her own for long periods. She never disturbed classroom activities and was usually not even noticed. Her school work, however, caused much concern.

Although Samantha was liked by fellow students and teachers, her parents noticed that her school achievements were well below her apparent potential and she began to fall behind in her academic attainment. She experienced difficulty in maintaining attention, was easily distracted and very disorganized in her school and home surroundings. Tasks would have to be repeated constantly and although she obviously heard the instruction, she was not really listening and could not therefore carry out the instruction.

She was extremely slow in starting what was required of her and equally slow in finishing. Because of the deterioration in her work, her confidence and self-esteem became very vulnerable and despite extra hours of work both in the classroom and at home, she made little or no progress. It was not surprising that Samantha was advised to repeat a year because of her poor grades. Her shy and quiet ways masked the warning signs of ADD. She and her parents were constantly reassured that she was only a slow learner and things would improve as she got older. As she created no problems in the classroom environment she was largely ignored.

Table 6.1 Core symptoms in ADHD

Poorly sustained attention/poor persistence of effort
- Easily drawn off task
- Bored quickly
- Loses interest and motivation

Impulsive/poor delay in gratification
- Must act now!

Hyperactivity/poorly regulated activity
- Excessive activity
- Situationally inappropriate activity
- Transitions difficult

Diminished rule-governed behaviour
- Failure to follow through on instructions
- Situationally inappropriate behaviour
- May include defiant behaviour

Table 6.2 Core symptoms in ADD

- Poor selective attention
- Poor sustained attention
- Poor interpretation of information
- Difficulty in starting or initiating tasks
- Difficulties in completing activities
- Daydreamer

TREATMENT FOR ADHD AND ADD

Help for the ADD/ADHD child and the family is best provided through a multimodal approach covering the medical, emotional, behavioural and educational needs of the child. Programmes include medication to help improve attention and reduce impulsivity and, if necessary, hyper-activity, training parents to understand ADD and be more effective managers. Counselling and training children in self-control and learning strategies, psychotherapy to help the demoralized child and other interventions at home and at school to enhance self-esteem and foster acceptance often prove critical to success. Treatment of the medical aspects of ADD is dependent upon ongoing collaboration between the prescribing paediatrician, teacher, therapists and parents. At Fairley House this seldom involves more than 2–3% of the children, but for this small number the results have been most encouraging.

Stimulant medication can be very effective in the treatment of both ADHD and ADD. Evidence confirms that these children respond to moderate doses by becoming more attentive and relaxed. The problem will not disappear overnight and so requires intensive treatment in mul-tiple areas. With appropriate help, improvement is apparent both at school and at home.

Research is now available to show the scientific foundation of medical treatment. If administered properly, to well-evaluated children, significant and meaningful improvement will occur in over 80% of ADHD children and slightly less in ADD children. Stimulants increase attentiveness, reduce distractibility and hyperactivity and improve overall academic and social functioning. A child who is appropriately medicated should never exhibit alarming changes in personality or mood. Most children on medication recognize that the medication must be working because they are no longer being reprimanded by the teacher, their handwriting has improved and they are now able to finish their homework within a much shorter time. Conflict with brothers and sisters also becomes far less of a problem.

The two main medications used throughout the world are methyl-phenidate (Ritalin) and dexedrine. They are both short-acting drugs, having an effect for a maximum of four hours. At least two doses are required for the school environment and a further dose may be necessary around mid-afternoon to counter any rebound reaction. The quick action makes it easier to observe the effect and adjust the dose as required. There are no withdrawal effects and the medication can be stopped safely at any time. Any side-effects are rare because of this action. However, the short action is really a mixed blessing. A longer acting drug would be preferable to accommodate the whole day's programme, but this has not been achieved by the pharmaceutical kingdom as yet. Sustained, regular, slow release of the medication over the course of the whole day would be ideal.

Dosage initially relies on weight, but should be modified depending on the subsequent response. This should only be done on medical advice and parents should not be encouraged to alter the medication. Follow-up visits are essential to monitor results. The medication should be given to cover the school week, Monday to Friday, but if the child cannot cope over the weekends or on holiday, it is not unreasonable to maintain the medication on a permanent basis.

There are few side-effects in most children taking Ritalin. The most typical problems, insomnia and loss of appetite, tend to disappear after a few weeks. Stomach aches and headaches are rarely significant and usually are only transient. Weight loss is not serious enough to be of medical consequence. Nevertheless, the Paediatrician should weigh the child regularly to record current state and weight gain. Effect on growth has been well studied and rarely occurs, and only with a high cumulative dose. Other non-stimulant drugs are available, but their effect is minimal. Many behaviours are wrongly attributed to the medication but when they arise they should be discussed with the consultant concerned.

The dosage should be modified until there is an optimal effect and the parent–teacher ratings of behaviour and side-effects should be reviewed regularly and the necessary adjustments made. There is no evidence that the medication leads to aggressive behaviour and there is no literature suggesting addiction for children or any greater risk of later substance abuse. Other groups of medication, e.g. the tricyclic antidepressants, are less effective in ADHD but can be used with a stimulant when associated anxiety, depression or severe mood swings are present, together with the ADD.

Intense educational input, counselling and behaviour modification programmes must accompany medical treatment. This requires a team approach and each member must define his or her strategy so that everyone is clear about what input is needed. The involvement of the parents is paramount and they should always know how the team is thinking.

A community education approach to make people aware of and understand ADD is important to improve the management and outlook of these children. Once identified, ADHD/ADD children are best managed by this multimodal approach. Good results are obtained when behavioural management programmes, educational interventions, parent training, counselling and medication are used together to help the child.

Parent support groups

Being told that your child has a specific learning difficulty which needs medical and educational input can come as a great shock to a family, no matter how carefully and sensitively the problem is explained. On the other hand, relief that a diagnosis has been made can be equally comforting, despite the nature of the difficulty. In both these situations, however, contact with other families may provide comfort in sharing similar experiences and several parent support groups have now been established to facilitate this. Groups now support a wide range of learning disorders and families with this problem have the chance of establishing contact with others similarly affected (Appendix 1 gives addresses). The support groups also help to advance understanding of the child's condition as well as providing more information and practical advice on management. All aspects of care can be enhanced in this way and we should all be working closely with them and supporting them in their endeavours.

Future research

As mentioned previously, research on the neurobiological basis of dyslexia is progressing. The reciprocal interactions between the various groups of functions (neurological, neuropsychological, cognitive) probably determine the way a learning disability is expressed clinically. It is important to analyse how medicine can interact with such a diverse and complex system as a cognitive disorder. Keeping the theoretical and clinical problems in mind, we need to evaluate the efficacy of medicinal and rehabilitative methods. For example, we might consider piracetam, a nootropic compound known for its learning and memory-enhancing properties. Discrepant results have been obtained in the USA, suggesting that piracetam's effect can vary over time as well as with different dyslexic populations. Further work in this area continues.

Newer and more sophisticated imaging techniques, e.g. magnetic resonance imaging (MRI), may prove useful in trying to find a neurological or anatomical basis for specific learning disabilities and variations in cerebral blood flow or metabolic activity might be instructive. So far this has not yielded convincing evidence.

The possibility of inheriting dyslexia and the inheritance of phonological processing characteristics are now well proven and genetic evidence of linkage has been recorded in dyslexic families. Associations between dyslexia and other disease processes, i.e. autoimmune disease, have already been reported and further associations will manifest themselves. There is still much to decipher in this exciting field.

References

Bakker, D.J., van Leeuven, H.M.P. and Spyer, G. (1986) Neuropsychological aspects of dyslexia. *Child Health Development*, **5**, 30–9.

Barkley, R. (1990) *Attention Deficit Hyperactivity Disorder*, Guilford Press, New York.

Cardon, L.R., Smith, S.D., Fulker, D.W. *et al*. (1994) Quantitative trait locus for reading disability on chromosome 6. *Science*, **266**, 276–9.

Connors, C.K, (1970) Cortical visual evoked response with learning disorders. *Psychopathology*, **7**, 416–28.

Snowling, M.J. (1995) Developmental dyslexia. *Current Paediatrics*, **5**, 110–13.

Appendix

The ADD/ADHD Family Support Group
c/o Mrs G. Mead
1a The High Street
Dilton Marsh
Nr Westbury
Wiltshire BA13 4DL
01373 826045
This group can offer a range of information and advice plus a list of self-help groups available around the country.

The National Learning and Attention Deficit Disorder Association (LADDER)
PO Box 700
Wolverhampton
WV3 7YY
A good source of information on AD/HD from across the world with a particular interest in medication and in adult sufferers of AD/HD.

The Hyperactive Children's Support Group (HACSG)
71 Whyke Lane
Chichester
West Sussex
PO19 2LD
This group has a special interest in therapies or treatments that avoid medication and can advise on nutritional approaches to AD/HD.

ADD Information Services
PO Box 340
Edgware
Middlesex
HA8 9HL
0181 905 2013
Fax: 0181 386 6466
Offer a wide range of books, videos and audio tapes for sale by mail order. Free information and advice is available on the phone and they also organize conferences across the country.

7   The School Counsellor

Vivienne McKennell

Far too often in the management of dyslexia the child is regarded as the sole focus of attention, whereas in reality they are part of a family, a community and are members of a specialist school. None of us functions in isolation. At times, there are stresses in all our lives which compound the difficulties we experience at work or in school. Equally, parents can be a very positive support providing they fully understand the nature of a child's difficulties. A therapeutic involvement with 'the worry lady' has not only lessened the stress and anxiety experienced by children, but has made them much more ready and eager to learn. Equally, being able to support and advise within the child's home has added an extremely useful and perceptive level of understanding to the management of specific learning disabilities.

P.G.

Case study

Rory did not like being dyslexic. It made him sad. It made his parents sad too; in fact, the only seemingly happy person in the family was Pam, Rory's high-achieving younger sister. Rory's competent and sympathetic class teacher despaired of getting to the root of his withdrawn behaviour and felt, despite all her efforts, he was working far below his considerable potential, as shown by the Educational Psychologist's report. In no way could he 'access the curriculum', nor participate effectively in the social activities of his peers.

After discussion with the Headteacher, I was asked to meet Rory to see if he might open up to me in a different situation from the busy classroom which he associated with failure. His parents' permission was sought and they greatly appreciated an opportunity for Rory to receive some help via a 'low key' approach, in preference to a formal referral to the local child psychiatric service. Discussion with the Headteacher, class teacher and Educational

Psychologist gave me a good picture of why everyone felt so concerned about Rory and I arranged to talk with him for half an hour in my room at school.

At first he was quite monosyllabic, staring at his feet and clearly hating being there. Gradually he started to tell me about his 'showy-off' sister, Pam, who seemed to get all the good things and how Dad liked her much better than him. It was easier when Dad was away on business, which he was a great deal, although it was then that his mother shouted at him, particularly when he did not do his home-work, which turned out to be most nights. Rory said he hated getting up for school each morning and would stay in bed until the last possible moment, by which time his mother was screaming at him and the day began badly even before he got to school to face fur-ther inevitable failures. I sympathized with Rory as to how sad he must feel at home and told him I would like to talk with his parents and see if we could try to make things a little easier for him.

Rory's parents eventually came to see me together, although it took a significantly long time to find a convenient appointment, as the father was always so busy. Within five minutes, his mother had burst into tears, saying she found Rory's behaviour terribly diffi-cult, particularly as she was on her own with the children so much. Was it any wonder she enjoyed her 'easy' daughter more? It became apparent that father blamed mother for Rory's dyslexia – 'She can hardly spell' – and he too made it quite clear that the only joy he felt in the home was from his daughter. Clearly there was much tension between the parents precipitated by the father's work demands and aggravated by the mother's problems with a child whom she perceived as a constant source of worry and irri-tation. Rory's guilt at being dyslexic and generally less able than his sister had made him sullen and even more difficult to handle. His depression fed his mother's depression and so a dreadful downward spiral of family dysfunction was taking place.

The next time I met the parents Rory came along too, with his sister. She was indeed a delightful child, who nevertheless complained that the mother spent 'hours' every night helping Rory with his homework and there was always shouting in the home which upset her, even though it was not directed at her. Rory was most surprised to hear this and to realize Pam also had her worries. Both children said how much they missed their father and how much nicer everything was when he was home. Further sessions with the parents resulted in the father reassess-ing his work priorities, cutting down his business trips to spend more time with the family. At school, Rory started to talk a little more to his teacher and one day after a concert, said he wished he 'could play the guitar like that'. The Head spoke with the parents about this and they were delighted that, at last, Rory had spontaneously shown an interest in something. Guitar lessons were arranged and, to everyone's surprise, Rory showed quite a talent and within the year was playing for the school assembly.

The old adage 'Nothing succeeds like success' is strikingly apt with the low self-esteem of dyslexic children. Success in one, even small, area can quickly generalize to the rest of their functioning; it is as if a 'light goes on' in their young lives. Socially Rory founds friends who admired, firstly, his guitar-playing but then him as a person and his happier self was able to concentrate on school work and use the myriad resources made available to him by his teacher.

I have related Rory's story at length although it is not particularly remarkable or indeed unusual – there are many children at the school weighed down by similar problems because it is a school where, by the very nature of their learning difficulties, the children are more vulnerable to family and environmental pressures.

The *Oxford English Dictionary* defines 'therapeutic' as 'curative, of the healing art'. This broad, umbrella term is helpful to understanding my role in the school team. I attempt to practise the well-tried theories of child psychiatry with particular reference to the needs of dyslexic children. I look at ways in which dyslexia may be an additional factor affecting the interaction between the children and their families. 'Specific learning difficulties' is extended into a wider concept of 'environmental dyslexia' to encompass the complex relationship between the child's social, emotional and educational world.

My role differs from that of counsellors who traditionally work only with the child in the school setting. Family therapists work, as their title suggests, with whole families. Psychotherapists work with individuals, either a child or an adult, and marital therapists treat couples. I try to work in an eclectic way, attempting to create a therapeutic 'safety net' for the child. Rory's story illustrates my function as the 'worry lady', willing to see whichever permutation of family members seems appropriate. Every child's needs are different and each case should be approached individually.

Because the school is the only social agency that sees a child every day, the class teacher's influence on, and knowledge of, an individual child is considerable. Nevertheless, there are inevitably constraints on a teacher's energies, a lack of privacy in the classroom, ever-increasing educational demands and frequently only the time to consider a child in a group rather than in an individual context. In a good school where there is a benign but structured approach, children can make enormous academic progress and a concern for pupils' emotional problems is established as part of the good teacher's role. Sometimes, though, however much effort is made at school, a teacher may feel 'stuck'; there seems to be something inaccessible in the child which the teacher has neither the time nor remit to deal with.

There may be a sense of a 'hidden agenda' which the child is bringing into school, making the educational input unavailable to them. The effect of this on a child with special needs is particularly damaging as these children already have a lower starting point than those in mainstream schooling. Of course, all children, like adults, have their 'off days' – perhaps after a particularly late night or when developing an infection. The wise teacher can distinguish between these 'off days' and what are ongoing intractable or even worsening behaviours. The class teacher may feel like the continuous butt of a child's anger or depression, without any explanation. Children can 'dump' negative feelings onto a teacher who then feels increasingly uncomfortable and impotent to help. Such children need a caring adult who has the time to listen and is not simultaneously juggling with the demands of the timetable and other children.

Case study

I was asked to see Malcolm because his anger after every weekend became a regular occurrence. Malcolm was a very mature 10-year-old who told me about the recent break-up of his parents' marriage and how every weekend he went with his younger brother to stay with their father. Malcolm knew that this left his mother sad and alone for the weekend and yet Malcolm desperately wanted to be with his father too. This sad conflict was compounded recently because the father's girlfriend, Anna, was always at his flat. 'She lives in Southampton, why does she always have to be there at the weekend?' Although Malcolm actually got on well with Anna there emerged a problem of keeping this secret from his depressed mother whom Malcolm correctly predicted would be devastated to know his father was involved in a new relationship. Malcolm's problems were worsened by his fears that his chatterbox younger sister might spill the beans to the mother. Malcolm's sense of betrayal of his mother and simultaneous loyalty to his father made the situation intolerable. With each parent he behaved maturely and responsibly but school was the only place Malcolm could let off steam and this he did in no uncertain terms to his poor unsuspecting teacher, after every access/contact visit!

No child should have to carry such a burden and Malcolm and his father came to see me together. Clearly Malcolm's mother was in need of support to get over the trauma of her divorce and weekly sessions with me helped her to begin to rebuild her life. In time she became emotionally strong enough to hear about her ex-husband's new relationship. Malcolm was relieved not only of his 'secret' but in knowing too that his mother was stronger and happier and that each parent was able to continue their new life independently whilst still being a loving parent to him.

It is important that the school creates an ethos for staff whereby members can admit 'I can't get any further with this child', acknowledging that reaching such a professional boundary is a mature decision rather than a weakness. By making an appropriate referral to the school therapist, the classteacher can be satisfied that the child will receive help at an intimate level which cannot be given in the classroom. Calling in another professional to throw light on what is hidden but problematic by looking at the family dimension enables a child to benefit much more fully from the programme the school has to offer. When I first became involved with Fairley House I was given an opportunity to meet all the staff and explain what I could offer and this in-service day helped to develop a sympathetic acceptance of a holistic approach to the children's problems.

Teachers need a sympathetic ear themselves because conscientious professionals all have a tendency to assume too great a responsibility and this creates stress. Stress, in its turn, makes people lose their perspective on problems and blocks the energies they need to deal with them. A good Headteacher is well aware of this danger and will protect staff from working beyond their own area of expertise, although boundaries can be gradually pushed back, as experience grows. Most schools have a support system, usually pyramidal in structure, with the Headteacher at the apex and the school therapist is available to offer the Headteacher support, too, when necessary.

The guidance of a professional who has the training and experience to help in the appropriate therapeutic management of a child can avert errors and provide welcome reassurance. Discussion between the school therapist and a teacher can avert crises and diffuse potentially volatile situations.

Andrea's mother had MS which was deteriorating rapidly. The day after Andrea told her mother about her teacher's well-meaning enquiries about how the family was coping, her irate mother phoned school saying Andrea had told her the teacher felt mother was no longer able to manage and Andrea might be taken into care. Such misunderstandings can easily happen around sensitive issues, particularly because a classteacher rarely has the time or privacy to go slowly enough to pick up a parent's point of view. Alice's mother sent a letter to say she would prefer Alice not to go on the class skating treat. The teacher's understandable reaction was of a gross injustice on Alice's behalf; the mother was being punitive and depriving Alice of a class reward. In a phone conversation with the mother it transpired that in fact Alice already went skating twice weekly and really would much rather have an extra art lesson, which she loved, by staying in school. Mother, in fact, was on Alice's side.

In their initial training, teachers regrettably receive very little help in working with parents, particularly in relation to emotional issues. One often hears teachers say 'We're not social workers', yet many teachers are 'naturals' and they do establish fruitful relationships with parents. For a few teachers this is an uncomfortable aspect of their work and they are relieved to have support and advice when this whole area is outside their previous experience. We know that in medical training, if young students are not given help and opportunities to talk about and clarify their feelings on suffering and death, they deal with those issues in a defensive way by becoming brittle and 'jokey'. Similarly, teachers require support and in-service training to empathize with parents and the relentless demands of family life. An aggressive mother who is always criticizing the school needs help, not condemnation, no matter how tiresome she may be.

There is every advantage in adopting a holistic approach to a child's needs, particularly when it is offered 'in-house'. Only then are we recognizing the many influences on children's ability to take advantage of the education on offer. A fragmented approach to children's problems often creates enormous difficulties, even competitiveness between professionals, and does nothing to help a child to feel supported by a network of concern. Bowlby's (1969) seminal research and his development of attachment theory have elucidated the function of the family as a secure base from which children can explore and develop. Byng-Hall (1994) asks why the principles of how family attachments influence security cannot also be applied to relationships between social systems (such as the school, the family and psychological services) which affect the child's security. Clearly, children feel more secure if they sense each group is supportive of the other; collaboration between adults is crucial for children.

Having discussed the value of complementing the school's work with the therapist's input and the merits of such input being provided 'in-house', let us now consider the broad categories of problems appropriate for referral.

- Behaviour disorder, e.g. aggression, nervousness, withdrawal, depression, confrontational children, withdrawal into fantasy.

Rudy was desperate for attention; both his parents had fulltime demanding jobs and they only met as a family at weekends, when they were exhausted and resented Rudy's 'childish' demands to play with him. At school, Rudy would use confrontational behaviour such as swearing or deliberately disrupting other children's work; even negative attention felt better than none at all.

Alex was so unhappy at home, so overcontrolled and felt so unable to have his wishes heard that his one escape was to retreat into a fantasy world of horror where his anger with his parents was expressed by writing almost psychotic horror stories and by secreting to his room 'video nasties' lent by adolescent 'friends'.

- Psychosomatic symptoms, e.g. bedwetting, soiling, stammering, involuntary tics (although the latter seem to be rarer nowadays), skin rashes, abdominal pain, vomiting, the child who is keen to establish himself as a victim. It is essential that referral about any of these symptoms is made only after the child has had thorough medical checks and no physical causes have been found.
- In contrast to the above point, children may be referred where there is some known constitutional cause, e.g. minor brain damage which creates an 'oddness'. This may be difficult to detect or define and consequently is sometimes overlooked.

Alan's father had been present at his birth. The hospital were short-staffed and when the newborn infant became distressed, the nurse had asked the father to go for oxygen as quickly as possible. In his panic and unfamiliarity with the situation, the distraught man brought an empty cylinder and the delay until a full one was found contributed to Alan's minimal brain damage.

- Obsessional states, often directly connected with too much psychological pressure, e.g. persistent handwashing or tying shoe laces again and again.

> Sandra was always the last to finish classwork, because she could never begin until her books and papers were, and remained, exactly parallel to the sides of her desk.

It will raise the level of awareness of children's emotional problems if referral decisions in a school can be made at the instigation of any of the multidisciplinary team involved with that particular child. Sometimes it may be the Headteacher who requests the additional help. In other circumstances, the referral may arise out of group discussion among concerned members of staff. Alternatively, it may be the parents who are aware of the facility I offer and request it for their child. In any event, parents' permission must be obtained, usually by the Headteacher.

The way this is discussed and the strength of belief in it is crucial to its success. It is essential that the referral to a therapist is seen by parents to stem from concern, never as a punishment or an end-of-the-line desperate measure. Certainly some parents find it more comfortable to talk with a non-teacher about intimate family details. It is often helpful to explain to younger children that the therapist is a 'worry lady', who can talk with them about their worries so that they will start to feel better and who is also someone good at keeping secrets. The point of referral in the child's school career is also important to note. It is, regrettably, not uncommon for children to be referred later than is desirable. Often a child may have reached the last year of primary school before staff acknowledge that he is very likely to encounter difficulties at the secondary school stage. A referral at this time means the child is coping with the not inconsiderable adjustments and anxieties of a school change as well as his precipitating problems. Clearly, the earlier the referral the better.

The therapist will have talked with the class teacher, the Headteacher and other relevant staff and had access to the child's file and records. The child might be observed in class at this point to note group behaviour. Reports of other involved professionals such as a Paediatrician, Speech and Language or Occupational Therapist will also be noted. The Educational Psychologist's report will provide a yardstick of the child's academic strengths and weaknesses. There is frequently an unusual discrepancy in this population of children between their performance and verbal scale results. Where a child shows poor verbal ability, particularly a younger child, I may find it helpful to provide some drawing materials or finger puppets to facilitate communication.

Talking with involved staff provides a 'feel' of the child and their difficulties. Many members of the team have counselling skills and the role of the Educational Psychologist, in particular, could easily overlap with mine. Boundaries have been made, however, because the children associate the Educational Psychologist with educational issues and with psychological testing. I can then be brought in as a 'dispassionate outsider' who, although made aware of the educational problems, is given space to look at other (i.e. home) factors which are influencing the child's attainment. Bowlby (1969) explained:

> Children, siblings, parents, class teachers, head teachers and others each have a distinctive perspective and favour a solution that commonly takes into account only a part of the problem ... the 'outside' professional has an opportunity to ... enable each of them to understand the viewpoint or expectations of others.

After the therapist's assessment has been made, a treatment plan will be drawn up. This needs to be flexible in terms of which family members are to be involved and also to take into account changing circumstances – a new baby, for example, can completely change the family dynamics the therapist is working with. If a family lives a long distance from where I practise, I see them in school; otherwise meeting on 'neutral ground' can be helpful.

Treatment may involve individual work with the child and/or one or both parents. If the child's behaviour is partly a result of marital difficulties, the therapist may decide to work on these and not see the child again. Sometimes family therapy, to include all members of the household, can be helpful, particularly when a child is being scapegoated and seen as the cause of all the family's troubles. In a session 'vicious or virtuous cycles of interaction become plain; ... the role of the professional is of mediator, clarifier and facilitator' (Bowlby, 1965).

Clearly, the main focus of the therapist's work centres around family relationships and how to enable family members to make these more comfortable. However, we must also acknowledge that it is unrealistic to hope there is a cure for everything somewhere 'out there' and that by bringing in more and more 'experts' the magic will be found. Regrettably, this is not always so. There are some very sad and unjust situations in this world which cannot be changed and for some families all we can hope to offer is support and understanding, so that the unbearable can become bearable.

Feedback and confidentiality

Another important part of the therapist's role is to liaise between school and home, to feed back, within the bounds of confidentiality, developments and changes so that school and home become closer in the common goal of helping the child. It is very reassuring for a child to feel that there is a benign concern for them from all the adults with whom they are in daily contact. Acceptance by staff that the therapist is part of the school team facilitates communication and, as noted earlier, such a structure moves away from the traditional fragmentation of services and helps to lessen the risk of the child as 'patient' moving from service to service with the attendant reinforcement of being 'a problem'.

An important part of a therapist's training is to recognize the importance of confidentiality in the therapeutic relationship, i.e. between therapist and patient, because it is only when the patient is able to feel total trust that they can begin to unburden themselves, perhaps for the very first time. Sometimes, even after one meeting, the therapist may gain a great deal of information about the family, some of which may be confidential, and this raises problems in relation to feedback to staff. It is clearly essential that reports and social histories should never be left lying around, nor should private discussions be held with open doors within earshot of passers-by. Such basic practicalities are not trivial; they are an essential part of professionalism.

As noted above, the therapist may become party to very intimate knowledge, which must be kept private and yet is clearly relevant to the child's management in school. A mother, for example, may have a drink problem. John's father had spent time in prison for tax fraud with all the stress and shame falling on the family. No wonder that, in school, John had suddenly become sullen and angry. Regrettably, issues of confidentiality are not, as a matter of course, part of teacher training and whilst most teachers are able to accept the concept in a mature way, and indeed at Fairley House are reminded formally of the issue at the beginning of each term, the withholding of information by the therapist can generate feelings of exclusion and anger. After all, the teacher is left 'holding the baby' and has to deal with all the difficult behaviour on a daily basis. However, management issues at school can be discussed with staff and, often with time, the parents may be encouraged to give their permission for confidential information to be passed on. This is a difficult area for all the adults involved and acknowledgement of the needs of each has to be worked out and respected.

Parents

Before meeting with parents I see the child alone. This puts 'meat on the bones' of the various reports, verbal and written, that have constituted the referral. It is also crucial that parents know I have actually met their child and can share, for example, their pleasure at his articulateness or alternatively, their despair with his constant fidgeting! After this initial interview with a child, I always telephone the parents to introduce myself and explain why I have been brought in and how I consider I might be of help. Otherwise parents may understandably become wary and think staff and the therapist are 'ganging up' on them. At this point, therefore, I always reassure parents of confidentiality both for the child – although with younger children this needs to be fairly flexible – and for the parents themselves. It is important, if the meeting is to be held in school, that a quiet room can be provided with comfortable chairs and no telephone or other interruptions; somewhere parents and children can feel safe and know that confidences will be respected and in no way overheard.

Initially, I always ask to see both parents together, as that in itself signifies the equal importance of each to their child's welfare.When parents live separately I see the custodial parent first, but always seek permission to speak with the 'absent' parent as soon as possible.

Let us now consider some of the demands on parents and how **their** role might be supported, because parenting can be a lonely task yet remains perhaps the most demanding many adults are faced with. What has gone wrong and why? Sympathetic and practical advice about management will have already been offered by staff, particularly by the Headteacher and/or the Educational Psychologist. Now the child needs to be considered in full context because children are more than school pupils from 9am to 4pm. Their personal and emotional behaviour needs looking at in conjunction with parents in a sympathetic, non-judgemental way.

Parents are the most important people in a child's life and they have an intimate knowledge of their child through closer association in the home long before and after the child begins and finishes school. Yet none of us can ever be a 'perfect parent', no matter how hard we try. Mistakes are inevitable and part of the human condition. This is why Winnicott's (1969) phrase the 'good enough mother' (and one might add 'father') is so releasing. Not surprisingly, many parents are filled with anxiety about the demands of the parental role and there is a need to support family life so that parents are enabled to carry out their role more effectively (McKennell, 1975). This is particularly true where children have specific needs because such children take a tremendous toll of parents' emotional resources. The child who has a difficult educational career also has parents who have had a difficult time in accepting their child's special needs. They have had to face repeated disappointments, guilt and failure; feelings experienced by most parents at some time or other, but here writ large and for public consumption. As a wise friend of mine once said, 'Why does everyone else's child get school prizes **and** play the violin?'

Despair with a child's behaviour at home may lead parents into defensive attitudes, difficulties in facing up to and admitting the truth and blaming the school for not doing its job properly. This may be aggravated because dyslexia is frequently hereditary and a parent may see their own mistakes and deficits being repeated in their child. Parents who themselves have similar problems to their child can simultaneously identify with and yet be contemptuous of those very difficulties which have caused them so much discomfort throughout their own lives. A dyslexic adult's problems with receptive and expressive language can make them appear suspicious and wary in discussion and this can present itself as apparent aggression.

When parents meet the therapist there are likely to be many initial anxieties stemming from their own childhood experiences of school and authority figures, particularly if they too had learning difficulties. They may also have had authoritarian parents with whom they never learned to negotiate; rational discussion may not be part of their experience in dealing with problems and they may now be panic-stricken with worries about their child. The interactions of their past and present, their inner and outer worlds, are what the therapist will be presented with initially and build on positively. It takes time and patience to surmount deeply entrenched attitudes and emotional pain and for parents to feel that, at last, here is someone they can trust and who will not condemn them for their mistakes and feelings of failure.

'The family is the most efficient and humane system of socialization we know. The continuous interaction between family and society means that when society is undergoing change, the family must respond likewise' (McKennell, 1975). It can be argued that the main need for a contemporary family is flexibility and a similar flexibility must be reflected in the response of those professionals coming into contact with today's families.

The social history

To gather the relevant information to enable the therapist to effect some change in the family, an oral social history is taken. The school has a very helpful family questionnaire which parents complete before a child's entry into the school. However, there is a world of difference between filling out a form and talking it through. Dale's mother and father, for example, had completed their form with an alarming list of negatives; Dale wouldn't sleep, eat or do his homework. He stole money, had no friends and was rude, swore at them and wet his bed – clearly a cry for help from desperate parents! However, in discussion with me, the parents painted a much more positive picture of their son. Dale was very helpful and caring to his infirm grandmother who lived with them. The material in the file therefore is helpful to give the therapist factual background information and is a valuable springboard into the first meeting with parents.

The social history is a way of gathering information so that we can look at the psychodynamics of the family. It is about parent–child interaction, not teacher–child or child–child interaction, because we need to know about the emotional environment in which a particular child is expected to develop. It is a means of collecting not just facts, but also impressions of emotional situations. It reveals the significance of issues parents consider to be important, of family relationships and of the strengths and weakness of family members. It is the fundamental tool of the therapist and fills the time of the first interview. Indeed, sometimes, because of the in-depth questioning and subsequent discussion, the social history can in itself be sufficient to unlock long-standing problems. This may be the first opportunity a parent has had to offload pent-up frustrations, anxieties and anger so that any further meeting may prove unnecessary. The history-giving itself has been sufficiently therapeutic.

It is important to get back to the very beginnings of a child's history, i.e. back to pre-birth. Was this child wanted and planned or 'a mistake' seen as precipitating a minefield of practical problems by being born to a couple who were not yet ready for parenthood and 'trapping' them into marriage? Were the pregnancy and birth complicated or easy? There appears to be a strong correlation between premature birth and subsequent dyslexia, although the dynamics of this link are still unclear. How might these experiences colour subsequent attitudes to the child and how does that compare with births of other children in the family? Already we can see how the earliest experiences can affect the parent–child relationship and they are important because difficulties in infancy can cause problems later, particularly in adolescence. After the birth how much support did the mother have? Was the father around? Or grandmother? Did the mother suffer a postnatal depression, thus complicating the early bonding process? Was there a series of unsatisfactory and ever-changing caretakers or au-pairs with English language limitations?

The social history then continues tracing a path through the 'milestones' of the child's development. Was feeding breast or bottle? Did the child feed well or was he a 'picky eater' or 'demanding'? There is some evidence that dysarthria and dyspraxia are related to difficulties in the fine motor control of the mouth and tongue so that in such cases, early feeding will be hampered, the caregiver will become frustrated and angry and feeding will be established as a time of tension. Were there any unusual factors, such as late or early language development, suggesting subsequent difficulties or strengths? Was there an over-emphasis on 'cleanliness' during toilet training?

The child's birth rank and gender can have a fundamental effect on a parent's relationship with their child. 'The responsible eldest', the youngest 'baby', the 'lonely only' and 'the middle child' are well documented. But we do not always recognize the effects of being the second boy when a much wanted daughter comes next or of being 'yet another' girl in a family of four daughters, where the father longs for a son to play football with. There are so many hidden factors which can influence the parent–child relationship and it is only with sensitive questioning that these may be brought to light, perhaps for the first time.

Having gleaned some insights into past development, we need to consider the present family situation. The permutations of influences and experiences on a child are infinite, but listed below are some of the most common categories which may be creating problems.

MARITAL PROBLEMS

Are there problems between the mother and father that make the child worried? Patrick's school work took a sharp downturn when his father was made redundant and he heard his parents' late night discussions about finances. In an interview with the therapist and his parents, eight-year-old Patrick blurted out that he feared they 'would have to live in cardboard boxes on the street because that's what happens to people who don't have any money'. Adults often fail to recognize that, just as strain and anxiety affect **their** concentration at work, the same holds true for children. If a child is worried about parents' rows or money problems, how can they concentrate sufficiently at school? Marital break-up now affects such large numbers of children that a separate section is given to this topic later in this chapter.

SEPARATIONS AND ASSOCIATED TRAUMA

Were any hospitalizations anticipated and prepared for or did the child wake up one morning and find that his mother had been rushed away in the night? Not surprising – they will not settle to sleep after that! Death is the ultimate separation and the loss of a much loved grandparent or even the family pet can create deep sadness and fearfulness for a child. Once there is a realization that loved ones can disappear, what reassurance have we that those remaining might not also disappear? 'And who would look after me then?'

Michael's mother was a tour operator and frequently abroad, as was his father on business trips. Michael's day-to-day care was in the hands of a much loved carer who had been with the family since Michael's birth. When Michael was eight, the carer decided to leave and for Michael this was an enormous and frightening loss of the one constant adult in his life. At school, he became weepy and 'clingy', resisting going out to play or leaving his classteacher for lessons with another teacher.

This type of 'third parent bereavement' is increasingly common and one which parents may find difficult to acknowledge as it touches on so many areas of guilt around who is in fact the most significant adult for the child.

ENVIRONMENTAL FACTORS

The effects of poor housing are obvious. Sharing a bedroom with a crying baby or having nowhere quiet to do homework are common examples. David's father was an airline pilot and his shift system necessitated a stressed mother frequently trying to hush a hyperactive ten year old so that father could sleep.

Frequent house moves are a problem for dyslexic children, who find adapting to change particularly difficult. Suzie's father was in the diplomatic service and had been moved many times. Not only was this difficult for Suzie but there were very apparent strains on her mother, who had to adjust constantly to unfamiliar cities and cultures where she knew no one and yet had to support her children into new schools and friendship groups.

MENTAL AND PHYSICAL ILLNESS IN THE FAMILY

Is there a close relative who has suffered from mental illness? Often there are fears this might resurface in one of the children and a parent may over-exaggerate any odd behaviour in their child to a point where a very ordinary problem may become reinforced and then become a real difficulty – a self-fulfilling prophecy. Rachel's father, who was living separately but nearby and saw Rachel frequently, had suffered a mild coronary a few years ago. Rachel knew that stress was bad for her father and so attempted to be very good when she was with him. Mother and school had to deal with all the 'held back' naughtiness of a naturally lively 11-year-old.

TRAUMATIC EXPERIENCES

Children can deal with surprising amounts of trauma if they have received adequate parenting and the parents themselves are coping in a sensible way; expressing their own distress, listening to the child's fears and placing the trauma in perspective. Margaret coped amazingly well when the family home was burned down. Sensible parents, who were supported by grandparents with whom the family were able to live, rode out the chaos and losses until a new home was eventually established.

THE 'PARENTAL CHILD'

A child may develop this quality when they have to take on the mantle of responsibilities too soon. A father constantly travelling abroad for weeks at a time meant Frank, aged seven, was expected by his rather feckless mother to be the 'man of the house' with all the resultant pressures on poor Frank. He would sleep in his mother's bed when his father was away and was perplexed and upset when he had to go back to his own room on his father's return.

Peter stayed awake each night listening to his parents' violent arguments, ready to rush downstairs and protect his mother.

Daisy became socially isolated and withdrawn and could not invite friends home after school because she never knew whether her mother would welcome them or react in an embarrassingly offhand manner. Unpredictability is particularly hard for dyslexic children; external routine helps contain their inner chaos.

THE 'PEACEMAKER' CHILD

Some children growing up in families where there is constant conflict take it upon themselves to be the 'peacemaker', the one who sees their role as keeping the family together by being ever good and helpful. Their own anger is never acknowledged for fear of causing further disruption. As children, they will poignantly have lost out on the normal fun and naughtiness of childhood and as adults they may become part of an abusive marriage where they tolerate far too much uncaring treatment because that is what is familiar to them.

PHYSICAL PROBLEMS

The danger with frequently ill children is that they may always be treated with 'kid gloves' and everything is attributed to the illness.

Sometimes parents who have had a sickly baby continue to treat their child as an invalid even when they have developed healthily after a shaky start. Many dyslexic children come into this category, because there is a link between birth trauma and/or postnatal complications and specific learning disabilities. Frequently parents' guilt at having a dyslexic child and the ongoing anxiety that the mother did something wrong, perhaps in pregnancy, can lead to overprotectiveness. It is a mechanism to keep at bay enormous anger and ambivalence. 'If I didn't spoil him, I'd kill him.'

Jake had severe scars on his arm from a car accident in which his mother was the driver. He would roll up his shirtsleeve and frighten other children in the playground. For a child with low self-esteem an increase in status is welcomed from any source! His mother's understandable guilt made her quite unable to chastise Jake about his behaviour although the reality was that, despite his disability, Jake was a nine year old needing structure and boundaries just like any other nine year old. By helping the mother with her guilt, she gradually began to accept this and was able to discipline Jake in an appropriate manner. Jake's anger with his disfigurement and his need to turn his terrifying experience into terrifying others diminished. He resumed more normal friendships with his peers and began to settle down to school work just as he had before his accident.

There are overweight children whose mothers so need to feed them that it is clearly the mother who needs help and support. More often than not, when the mother is able to develop constructive goals in her life, the child is less stifled and begins to develop in a healthier way. Paul's mother had a series of miscarriages over eight years before Paul was born. It was hardly surprising she found it difficult to 'let go' of her 'special' child.

SIBLINGS

The significance of birth rank and gender has already been mentioned. There might be a frequently ill sibling with whom parents have to spend a great deal of their time.

Henry, a sensitive 8-year-old, was full of conflict and guilt concerning his severely asthmatic little brother, Tim, who often had to be rushed into hospital as an emergency. Henry picked up his parents' worries for the younger child and spoke with them sympathetically about Tim. At the same time, the limited resources and needs of an 8-year-old in his own right made Henry feel furious with Tim for absorbing so much parental attention. The parents were encouraged to talk with Henry and explain that for them, too, it was a dilemma and they had to prioritize their time, but understood how 'left out' Henry often felt. For Henry himself, it was a relief to know that his negative feelings towards Tim were understandable and indeed accepted. He felt less guilt and less need to oversentimentalize his concerns for Tim and was less aggressive in school whenever someone in his class received any of the attention he so desperately craved.

Sometimes a parent will spend an inordinate amount of time with the dyslexic child helping with homework. This is understandably resented by siblings, whilst the dyslexic child's resentment is because they miss out on 'fun' time with parents; prime time is always homework time.

EDUCATIONAL PRESSURES

There may be strong parental and/or family expectations and traditions. Mother may be overambitious for her child because she herself is underfunctioning and regrets her own lack of higher education. She may well feel a need for her child to show the world she can 'at least' be a successful mother and produce bright children. Whatever the reasons, expectations beyond a child's ability will invariably lead to behaviour problems. This is where discussion with the Educational Psychologist can be helpful. The definitions 'above average' or 'high average' will have been carefully explained to parents and the child's test scores put in the perspective of the general population. It may take a long time before the child's potential is completely understood. Parents' understanding may be blocked by difficulties with the technicalities, but also with resistance to accepting the true picture. It is very painful for parents to hear that their child is less able than they had hoped and it is sometimes helpful for the therapist to raise this issue again after liaising with the Educational Psychologist. In the long term, it can only be beneficial to the child when unrealistic educational pressures are lifted and parents helped to accept the child's strengths rather than focusing on the areas where they are less able.

CULTURAL DIFFERENCES

The Commission for Racial Equality (1989) has pointed out 'There is no "best" way to bring up a child and consequently professionals must be flexible in eliciting information so that it is not processed through the perspectives and values of the predominating culture'. Nevertheless, the fundamental issues around parenting are universal and, given an acceptance of cultural differences, the need for support and compassion transcends all boundaries.

SELF-ESTEEM

Dyslexic children frequently suffer from low self-esteem, which is itself aggravated by the social and educational problems associated with their special needs. Much research highlights this circularity, e.g. Pumphrey and Reason (1991). Motivation is linked to confidence and confidence in turn leads to a 'feel-good factor'. There is no point in applying the epithet 'could try harder' to a child who has neither the will, the courage or energy to face new challenges. The longer the child has struggled with the cumulative effects of failure, the harder it is to restore self-esteem and the earlier a referral for emotional help, the better.

Siblings at mainstream schools may tease a dyslexic brother or sister cruelly. Parents, also, may have their self-esteem shattered by having a dyslexic child. At each stage of schooling, they will be faced with difficult and painful decisions which most other parents do not have to consider. Their home life may be under constant strain because of the child's behaviour. Frequently, one parent blames the other for being the 'cause' of the child's problems – 'It's your side of the family who cannot spell' – and the marriage, too, may become fragile. This in turn causes anxiety for the child with further deteriorating behaviour. My task is to support families so that they themselves become strong enough to build up their child's self-esteem. Positive changes in family dynamics can enable a shift in the child's perception of themselves and subsequently perceptions of them by their family – an interactive process which can then continue to spiral upwards.

Bullying

Low self-esteem means dyslexic children easily become victims of bullying and find it difficult to stand up for themselves because they frequently feel that they deserve unfair treatment. Sometimes it is helpful for me to see the bully and victim together. The aim is to help the bully to at least begin to be sensitized as to why they make the other child so unhappy. The victim is encouraged not only to be more assertive but also to understand how they may irritate or provoke other children.

Divorce

In 1994, close on one in three marriages in the UK ended in divorce. This means an enormous number of children have to cope with the pain of family break-up. One positive outcome of this statistic is that the sheer weight of numbers involved has led to a parallel expansion in research and clinical practice in this field, so that there is now a broad knowledge of relevant theory and treatment (Cockette and Tripp, 1994). It is essential to refer children who appear to be showing distress relating to family break-up as early as possible, because the appropriate expertise is available and the earlier the intervention, the better. Mediation services where the welfare of the child is paramount or a counsellor/ therapist with experience in this area of work can help protect the long-term mental health of the child.

Divorce is a process, not an event, and it is likely, therefore, that the child and other family members have been suffering for a long time. The divorce rate in marriages with a 'handicapped' child is higher than the average and there is no doubt that dyslexic children can be extremely difficult to live with, especially when there is a hyperactive element in their behaviour. In some families the actual decision to separate can be a relief from ongoing discord. But, as in any crisis, human beings may regress emotionally at such times and this applies to adults as well as children. Thus, for many children there is no safety net of a well-functioning adult at this time to protect them from the chaos and pain all around. Dyslexic children are particularly vulnerable to confusion and stress and help therefore may be most efficiently directed at supporting the adults so that they can adequately nurture the children.

We know that children, even from a very young age, often feel it is their fault that their parents have split up. 'If I had been gooder,' said five-year-old Nicky, 'Daddy would have stayed in my house.' Often dyslexic children are aware that they have disappointed their parents' expectations. They may hear parental rows about their school-work with (usually a father's) reluctance to face the problem and the financial implications of getting appropriate help. The type of programme which a specialist school offers is expensive and a sensitive child may suffer enormous guilt if parents are paying and a family holiday or a new car has to be sacrificed.

Darren was in tears about the long hours his father worked because he assumed they were to pay for his school fees. Father was in fact a workaholic and had been like this long before Darren came to the school. But Darren's misunderstandings had led him to feel tremendously pressured to do well at school and the distress which this caused him had compounded his already considerable educational difficulties. An opportunity for Darren to talk with his father lifted a huge weight of responsibility from his young shoulders.

Nevertheless, there are many instances where school fees are a great strain on family finances and the attendant pressure on children needs to be faced, painful as it is.

Understanding what is actually happening helps too. Retrospectively, many children complain they were never told what was going on around them. Ideally the child should visit the new accommodation of the non-custodial parent as early as possible. What will his father or mother eat? Have they got a real bed to sleep in? Parents are often amazed that children can worry about them. Access arrangements, or 'contact' as it is now called since the 1989 Children Act, is often where parents continue marital battles. Mother says 'No, you can't see Johnny on Sunday because he is invited to a birthday party'. Father, equally damaging, fails to pick up the child on time or, worse, never appears at all. Many fathers give up contact because of the distress caused by repetitive psychological loss of their children after each contact visit, particularly when faced with what lawyers call 'a mother's implacable hostility'. Research shows that what affects children most in divorce is the process by which the couple part and the degree of ongoing conflict. It is the high-conflict families who create disturbances in their children and the most distressed children are the ones who are made the focus of parental battles.

Continuity of care and concern for children is crucial. Adults can have an ex-house or an ex-job, but they cannot have 'ex-children'. Yet so often this happens because, without help, the difficulties may be too great for a parent to retain any nurturing links. During family break-up school can be a 'safe place' providing stability and continuity for a child. The teacher (although dependent on parents for updating information) can support a child on a daily basis through emotional chaos. A sympathetic school will help children with organizational problems, reminding them where they are going after school that day. Teachers can also be tolerant about lack of homework, etc. when they know what is going on. It is essential that a three-way information process is maintained between the two parental homes and school. Again, where parents are living apart, it is essential for the school to know the address and telephone number of the non-custodial parent, who may then also be invited to school events.

Children need to know when they will next see their parent after saying 'goodbye'; dyslexics are lost without regular routine and even very young children can be given a sense of time by marking days on a calendar. Brief contact with an absent parent is insufficient; the child ideally needs 'prime time' and enough of it to absorb information in what rapidly becomes a less familiar environment because these children, almost by definition, have poor listening skills and if intervals between visits are too long, they find it much harder than others to 'pick up the threads'. Children often behave badly after a contact visit because their sense of loss has also been rekindled and this may be misinterpreted by the resident parent as the absent parent 'spoiling' or unsettling the child. Support and explanation are needed if further visits are not to be curtailed – a common reaction. Custodial parents, and statistically this is still more likely to be the mother, can be very angry if, as often happens, they are responsible for reading practice, dental visits, etc., whilst the absent parent only does fun things at the weekend. This can lead to abuse of the absent parent and to greater acrimony, thus lessening the chance of the children effectively 'keeping' both parents.

Inconsistency about homework is a major problem for the dyslexic child with divorced parents. Books and resources always seem to be in the wrong house. If homework is not done, parents may blame each other and use it as yet another source of conflict. Any difficult behaviour may be put down to 'being just like your father' with consequent confusions for the child about identity and self-esteem. The very areas where dyslexic children cope badly, e.g. being disorganized or forgetful, may be the very shortcomings which initially irritated a spouse about their partner and when seeing a mirror image of these attributes in the child on a daily basis it requires a great deal of maturity for a parent to 'hold their tongue'. Children need to be helped to accept their 'bad' parent as a human being with strengths and weaknesses.

Because the UK has the highest rate of remarriage in Europe, we have large numbers of stepfamilies with all their potential complications and their need to be 'flexi-families'. But dyslexics are not flexible, this is one of their problems and so a non-biological parent may find it particularly hard to accept a dyslexic child, who may be uncooperative, tense and uncommunicative.

Clearly, the second half of the 20th century has seen enormous social changes and parenting has had to adapt. As traditional role boundaries become eroded, so the stereotypes of maternal and paternal behaviour need to be challenged and laid to rest (Wolfendale, 1992). Indeed, the adults in families nowadays may not both be the biological parents, they may not be married, they may not be of the same ethnic origins and may be of the same gender. However, because child rearing is so demanding, there is no doubt that it is almost always easier to share the task between two adults who can give each other mutual support.

FATHERS

In most cases women are still the primary caregivers to children and so to help fathers be more involved in their children's lives is a vital contribution that has different, but equally important, significance for daughters and sons.

Stephen was very worried about the forthcoming summer holiday when Daddy, whom he did not live with, was taking him and his brother to Italy. All Stephen wanted to do there was to play on the beach with his surfboard – his current favourite hobby. Daddy, a driving businessman, on the other hand, saw the summer holidays as an opportunity for him to make an impact on Stephen's schoolwork, which he felt was too lax when Stephen was at home with his mother. All poor Stephen could do was cry to his distraught mother and say he didn't want to go away with his father. I set up a meeting in school for Stephen to try to tell his father what was troubling him. Dyslexic children need extra time and space to state their problems because they cannot formulate and express ideas as quickly or fluently as other children. Stephen and I met therefore to 'plan an agenda' so Stephen could explain his distress and really communicate to his father what would constitute a 'fun' holiday. The Headteacher spoke with the father about how much reading practice was really necessary and gradually the father's anxieties about Stephen's education lessened. The pressures on Stephen became less and paradoxically, he was 'freed up' to concentrate on his school work and began to do very well in class.

We need to ask why the father is so important, when so many children live nowadays with their biological mothers. Indeed, the father's role in child development has only recently become subject to research and is still controversial (Lewis and O'Brien, 1987). The plight of 'absent' fathers in marital break-up has already been noted but, whether resident or not, their importance cannot be over-emphasized. The effect on a child's school attainment, particularly boys' reading, can be quite remarkable when a father becomes involved.

Psychoanalytic perspectives include Freud's theories of the Oedipus and Electra complexes including his belief in the father as the role model for the son and a 'love object' for the daughter. For Jung (1983), the father represents 'the spiritual', a figure connecting the child to values and ideas. Fathers also provide a connection between past and present. 'The image of the elder telling all he knows to the younger is a compelling one' (Samuels, 1985). More recently the influence of feminist ideas has challenged traditional beliefs and led to a complex but interesting debate beyond the brief of this chapter. Suffice it to say here that the more caring adults there are surrounding a child who know him intimately, the better. As one American paediatrician commented, 'A parent is a terrible thing to waste'.

Summary

This chapter has attempted to explain the advantages for school, family and the child of having an 'in-house' therapist attached to the school. It is via our children that society perpetuates its values and culture. For this and for straightforward humanitarian reasons, we must ensure that we use all the knowledge and skills at our disposal to protect and nurture the mental health of the next generation.

FOR THE SCHOOL

At a time of ever-increasing demands on staff, the school can gain by being able to call on a complementary area of expertise. The school can be seen as a wheel in which the spokes are different specialisms, all interdependent and reporting back to the Headteacher so as to provide maximum help for the child. The school therapist sheds light on the previously unknown dimension of a pupil's family background so that emotional blocks are released and educational attainment and management in school are enhanced.

FOR PARENTS

Parenting is arguably one of the most important tasks in society, but one for which we receive no training. Rapid social changes make it increasingly difficult for parents to fulfil their role, particularly when there are the added strains of a child with special needs. Home influences on educational attainment are paramount and therefore it is sound logic to support parents' self-esteem and confidence in their nurturing skills so that they can carry out their role more effectively.

FOR THE CHILD

When a child is sent to a specialist school for a period of intensive remedial help, the effort will be wasted if tension and stress block access to
the curriculum. The therapist can provide a bridge between the two
major influences in the child's life – home and school; a safe haven in
which to offload anxieties and make sense of what is often experienced
as pressure and chaos.

References

Bowlby, J. (1965) *Child Care and the Growth of Love*, Penguin, Harmondsworth.
Bowlby, J. (1969) *Attachment and Loss*, Vols 1 & 2, Hogarth Press and Institute of
Psychoanalysis, London.
Byng-Hall, J. (1991) *The Application of Attachment Theory to Understanding and
Treatment in Family Therapy*, Tavistock Publications, London.
Cockette, M. and Tripp, J. (1994) *The Exeter Family Study*, University of Exeter
Press, Exeter.
Commission for Racial Equality (1989) *From Cradle to School: A Practical Guide to
Race Equality and Childcare*, CRE, London.
Jung, C.G. (1983) *The Zofinga Lectures*, Routledge and Kegan Paul, London.
Lewis, C. and O'Brien, M. (eds) (1987) *Re-assessing Fatherhood: New Observations
on Fathers and the Modern Family*, Sage, London.
McKennell, V. (1975) Family life education – the role of the nursery/infant
teacher. MA dissertation, University of Southampton.
Pumphrey, P.D. and Reason, R. (1991) *Specific Learning Difficulties (Dyslexia)*,
NFER-Routledge, London.
Samuels, A. (ed.) (1985) *The Father*, Free Association Books, New York.
Winnicott, D.W. (1969) *The Child, the Family and the Outside World*, Penguin,
Harmondsworth.
Wolfendale, S. (1992) *Empowering Parents and Teachers*, Cassell, London.

8 *The remedial teacher*

Patience Thomson

The job description

The contribution to the remedial function by the classteachers, Speech and Language Therapists and Occupational Therapists is clearly documented elsewhere in this book. The role of the remedial teachers themselves is also a key part of the overall picture and needs to be described in some detail. It will be apparent that some part of their role as defined in this chapter is specific to an environment such as Fairley House, which is specialized and which involves the cooperation and interdependency of a multidisciplinary team. Other aspects, such as remedial techniques, are more general in nature.

The remedial teachers are expected to have responsibility for a caseload where the pupils' specific reading, spelling and written language problems are identified and appropriate programmes are drawn up. They see the pupils on their individual caseload, mostly on a one-to-one basis but also in small groups where appropriate. They are responsible for producing termly work plans and reports on individual children receiving remedial teaching for school records, for LEAs and for parents. They must at all times liaise with the Occupational Therapists and Speech and Language Therapists so that an informed and holistic approach can be adopted by both therapist and remedial teacher and due cognizance be taken of the educational needs of the pupils. They must keep in close touch with classteachers so that the remedial teachers are aware of pupils' performance in the classroom. They also work with the classteachers in the classroom as a team in appropriate lessons.

In addition they need to maintain close contact with parents, particularly in relationship to homework, organization and management strategies.

It is also expected that the remedial teachers should foster and develop areas of interest which can be shared with staff on INSET, or Study Days.

The remedial teachers have a group responsibility to ensure that the remedial programme devised for each child is appropriate and coherent and that it is regularly updated and revised. This extends to further responsibility for the administration of standardized reading, comprehension and spelling tests throughout the school and for the interpretation of the results.

Flexibility is the hallmark of the remedial teachers' trade. For some periods of the day they will work in partnership with the teacher in the classroom. Most of their time will be spent teaching small groups or individual lessons. In these they will address the specific difficulties of particular children, plugging any gaps, forging links between the various strands of remedial input and teaching the personal learning strategies, or study skills, which will enable the individual child to access the curriculum independently.

Close links are maintained with the senior Speech and Language Therapist over the content of the oral language skills lessons. In these sessions children learn to express their ideas verbally, often using tape recorders. In this way listening and communication skills are fostered. Organization and sequencing ability can also be developed. These sessions can support work in the classroom if, for instance, topic-related subjects are chosen for debate. The exercise then becomes more meaningful for the child.

The remedial teachers collaborate with the Occupational Therapists in devising individual schedules of work for children who need to improve their visual tracking skills or their letter formation and handwriting. Body posture will also be monitored. Presentation of work on the page may be a problem for the child with poor spatial skills.

The senior remedial teacher establishes the content of the structured, cumulative, phonics-based spelling programme. At Fairley House an in-house diagnostic test has been devised so that the children can be regularly tested to see if they have absorbed the rules and spelling patterns which they have been taught. The remedial teachers analyse the results of the diagnostic tests and ascertain which children need extra help in spelling and in which specific areas.

In mainstream schools with a remedial department, the remedial teachers often concentrate in individual lessons on improving the dyslexic child's reading competence, spelling and writing skills. They usually follow a structured, cumulative programme such as those suggested by Hornsby and Shear (1994), Augur and Briggs (1992), Miles (1992) and Cooke (1993). More rarely, problems in mathematics are addressed.

In a specialist environment, reading, spelling and written language skills can with advantage be taught throughout the school as a daily group activity, rather than in weekly individual sessions. This means that the content of the remedial teachers' individual programmes with the children can be redefined and this brings bonuses in terms of more freedom to target broader issues or address particular areas of difficulty.

One of the major problems with any remedial work involving written language is that skills can improve impressively when the child is in the one-to-one situation, but do not readily transfer to the classroom. Handwriting and spelling are especially vulnerable, with children forgetting the good practice and the rules which they have so painstakingly learnt with their remedial teacher when they come to use them 'for real' in class in their topic work or in their creative story writing. If the remedial teachers are also involved in the classroom, so that they can monitor how the child performs there, this gap can be bridged.

The remedial teacher's caseload is carefully selected to match particular teaching skills and personalities to appropriate pupils. It should be borne in mind that the one-to-one teaching situation may present the chance for an individual child to confer, confide or confess and this window of opportunity should be left open.

In all areas of basic literacy and numeracy, the remedial teachers can focus on areas of personal need. Children will be following an appropriate structured phonics programme in their group. The remedial teacher can personalize the phonic knowledge the children have acquired in group lessons by teaching them a related vocabulary which focuses on their particular interests, whether they be football, fishing or dinosaurs. If a child has failed to understand a particular concept or learn a spelling pattern or even if a child has been absent through sickness, the remedial teacher can find a wide variety of ways to reinforce input from the classroom without boring repetition. Depending on the interests and ability of the child, crosswords, word searches, rhyming games, mnemonics, quizzes and appropriate computer programs can all be used creatively to help the child to grasp and fully internalize a spelling rule or pattern which is proving difficult. The regular diagnostic spelling tests, which have been developed in-house to relate specifically to the school's phonics programme, identify immediately which types of words are creating problems for an individual child. This information is invaluable to the remedial teacher, who can target specific areas of weakness. They can also ensure that there is no duplication or omission within the structure of the remedial provision.

Individual education plans (IEPs)

Within the remedial department there is a wide range of options available. An appropriate plan will be drawn up each term for individual pupils, having regard to priorities. A child may have weaknesses in several areas, but these cannot all be addressed concurrently without overloading the programme. A balance must be maintained, because the children still need enough lessons weekly in the classroom to fulfil the requirements of the National Curriculum syllabus.

At the beginning of each term, the multidisciplinary team, which includes the Speech and Language Therapists, the Occupational Therapists and the remedial teachers, must draw up the individual education plans (IEPs) for the whole school. The Headteacher, the Educational Psychologist, classteachers and parents may also have views and sometimes particular requests which need to be taken into account. Senior members of the remedial team will have the duty to ensure that the children for whom they have been given overall responsibility are receiving an appropriate range of remedial help. All pupils receive standard remedial provision in reading, spelling, maths and oral language in small groups. Of these, reading alone is taken by individual members of staff while in the other sessions two members of staff will team-teach.

Specific remedial provision is provided according to current need by the different specialists, including the remedial teachers, in a one-to-one or small group context. It will include several, but not all, of the following at any one time.

- Written language and creative writing.
- Study skills.
- Touch typing and laptop skills.
- Extension reading group or maths in addition to the scheduled daily group lessons.
- Occupational therapy, including work on gross and fine motor skills and visual perception. This may be done individually, or in a group 'motor' class.
- Handwriting, under the supervision of the Occupational Therapist.
- Speech and language therapy including articulation, listening skills, vocabulary and language structure.
- Social skills, for children with inappropriate social behaviour.
- Art therapy for children who have poor self-image, cannot take risks and find interpersonal relationships difficult.

It may also be arranged for a teacher in a curriculum subject like music or design technology to give 'special' attention to a child. This can build a useful platform for success.

An integral part of the IEPs is the detailing of current strengths and weaknesses and a precise description of the immediate goals for that term.

One-to-one remedial sessions

One-to-one sessions are particularly useful for extending written literacy skills. The less imaginative children can be encouraged to experiment and explore. It is helpful to allow them to try to express their ideas through trial and error in a more private situation, unencumbered by fear of disapproval or competition from their peers. On the other hand, naturally creative and imaginative children, whose minds race ahead of their pens and who teem with bright ideas which they cannot express coherently, can be helped in individual sessions to organize and rationalize their thoughts. This can be done in note form, sometimes using the word processor or through the spider diagrams and mind maps suggested by Buzan (1993), so that the final written exercise has structure and form. Punctuation and style can also be discussed in more depth and the child's working written vocabulary extended. Draft work from the classroom can be brought to the remedial teacher, often saved on the laptop word processor. More time can be spent on revising, editing and proof-reading the text than would be available if this had to be left to the busy classteacher to complete in lesson time.

Preempting problems

Often the remedial teacher can preempt problems. The curriculum, including the topic subjects, is established at the beginning of term. The remedial teacher can therefore select and preteach, for example, the relevant vocabulary from the topic work or the new concepts in maths which will almost certainly cause problems for a particular pupil. The child then recognizes in class what the teacher is talking about, feels less threatened and is less likely to lose the thread of the lesson. This can be particularly useful for children whose receptive language skills are impaired. They may have poor auditory recall and be unable to listen to and comprehend immediately any concept outside their previous knowledge and experience.

Certain children pose special problems and may benefit particularly from individual tuition. Cohen (1994), writing about children with attention deficit hyperactive disorder (ADHD), states:

> Children with biologically based attentional problems typically perform much better on a one-to-one basis than they do in a group situation. Group settings are more stimulating and these youngsters may not have the physiological mechanisms to manage this. In addition, one-to-one settings tend to be emotionally safer, more secure and structured than group settings. Thus, an individualized

tutoring or clinical situation may not elicit the typical behaviour evident in group settings.

The needs of hyperactive and attention-deficit children can create a dilemma. It could be arguable that their best chance of acquiring basic literacy and numeracy skills, and in particular effective study skills strategies, lies in giving them the maximum number of one-to-one sessions possible. There is, however, great danger in removing them too often from the classroom. Not only may they be marginalized within their peer group, but eventual reintegration into mainstream education will be far more difficult if their daily timetable has focused unduly on individual sessions. remedial support must include strategies for learning to work in group situations, for focusing attention and screening out distractions. This may well be as important a priority as improving basic skills. Close consultation with the Educational Psychologist and the Paediatrician will help to establish the important guidelines for the identification and management of attention deficit hyperactivity disorder or ADHD (Barkley, 1990).

Metacognition

The remedial teachers, because they see the children individually or in small groups, acquire a detailed knowledge of their personalities and preferences and the pattern of their difficulties. This can be used to help them analyse their learning processes.

Dyslexic children are often incapable of crossreferencing areas of knowledge. They cannot easily generalize from the particular, establish stable systems of reference, perceive connecting factors or screen out irrelevant cues when fact finding. All these skills can be taught in small group situations, but some one-to-one intensive help may be needed initially.

The concept of 'metacognition' and the need to teach cognitive skills has recently been highlighted, in particular through the work of Feuerstein in Israel and others elsewhere (Lebeer, 1995). It entails giving children more understanding and control of the learning process. Hardman and Beverton (1993) have written about the development of 'metadiscoursal' skills, which refer to the children's ability to verbalize orally to the teacher and to their peers in class what they discover as they learn. This improves their ability to make sense of incoming information, to build on it and to draw worthwhile conclusions. The task of the remedial teacher is to foster the children's ability to evaluate the relevance of incoming material, to screen out the unnecessary, to learn what is important and to relate it to what they know already. Some children may accomplish this naturally but it has often to be specifically taught to dyslexic children.

Remediation through information technology

Considerable remedial time and effort will initially be spent helping the children to form the handwritten letters of the alphabet and to space them properly. However, even with much practice and guidance some children will struggle to produce a neat script and will quickly tire in the process. For them, handwritten work is more a physical chore than an opportunity for self-expression and communication. This is particularly true of dyspraxic children with poor motor skills, who are described in Chapter 4 and elsewhere in this book.

Information technology can be an important element in reestablishing confidence and enhancing self-esteem and has a wide range of uses within the remedial programme. Anyone who has ever drafted an important letter, report or script longhand, read it, had it typed out and read it gain, will recognize that satisfactory feeling of being able to distance oneself when the neat printed page replaces the original hand-written version. Handwritten work may be poorly presented on the page with some words partially illegible. Corrections look messy. These aspects distract the reader and detract from the content. Immediately the text is printed it looks more 'professional', more convincing, and is easier to evaluate. If this is true generally, how much more so for dyslexic individuals, with their weak spelling and their often uneven, poorly spaced, ill-formed handwriting. Judgement will already have been passed by the reader before the content is absorbed.

The dyslexic who is competent to use a word processor efficiently, who can touch type, access a spell check and revise the text is at a considerable advantage. Word processors afford the opportunity to improve and edit work and still produce an impressively neat final copy. Keyboarding reinforces kinaesthetically the phonic patterns in words, especially if this aspect is reinforced by the teacher. Dyslexic children may not easily see or hear the similarity between the words 'match', 'catch' and 'patch', but will recognize that they are using the same keys in the same order for all but the initial letter of each word. A built-in thesaurus is more useful in many ways than a dictionary, providing exciting alternatives. Key in 'fat' and you can access 'corpulent', 'obese', 'plump', 'overweight', 'massive' or 'elephantine', all of which can be transferred to the text at the touch of a key. No copying is required. Computers and word processors do not criticize, they have no memory of past errors, they encourage experiment and are conspiratorial in allowing mistakes to be covered up or erased without being made public. They also foster concentration, can give immediate feedback (as when the spell check bleeps), supply built-in selections of pictures to illustrate text and produce pie charts and graphs which look highly professional. They facilitate the power to impress, which is very important for the dyslexic child.

Dyslexic children are often comparatively computer literate and have considerable flair for information technology. They will be better able to cope with secondary school assignments if coursework can be done on a word processor. They may also have an area of superior expertise which will genuinely impress their classmates, the staff who teach them and family at home. Later on such competence will make it easier to find satisfying employment in adult life. There can be little doubt that spending time, money and energy on a serious commitment to information technology is a good use of both human and financial resources. The 'fun' element of learning is stressed and permanently useful skills acquired. It is important that the individual remedial teachers have the training and expertise to develop these skills in their one-to-one sessions.

Intransigent failure

It would be unreasonable to claim that any specific remedial programme offered is uniformly successful. While some children's progress may be remarkable and that of others satisfactory and acceptable, there remains a very small, hard core of pupils whose lack of improvement in the basic skills of literacy and maths remains a cause for considerable concern. The usual remedial strategies have not worked. Other approaches must be adopted if these children are not to sense that, even after transfer to a specialist school offering intensive support and remediation, their performance once again compares unfavourably with that of their classroom peers.

Careful screening is necessary through the regular analysis of in-house tests and by creating opportunities for discussion at staff meetings if incipient problems are to be identified at an early stage. Standardized reading, spelling and maths tests, used twice a year, provide useful data if they are entered on a database which then automatically records progress, lack of progress or, very occasionally, regression. Once an area of real concern has been established, options for rectifying the situation must be urgently considered.

READING EXTENSION GROUP (REG)

The purpose of establishing a reading extension group (REG) was to provide an alternative approach for those individuals whose reading skills were not improving satisfactorily within the standard provision offered in the school. The degree of retardation, the age of the child and the verbal score on the Wechsler Intelligence Scale for Children (Wechsler, 1991) were all factors in the decision to intensify the level of remedial help for a particular pupil.

Each REG meets three or four times a week. The teacher present acts as a facilitator and does not intrude as a teacher. The children themselves monitor their own progress, sometimes through timed testing of reading accuracy and speed. They encourage each other to attempt more ambitious passages in a graded reading programme and to experiment without fear of ridicule. They also play suitable reading games and use the computer. It is a therapeutic session, where these pupils can openly discuss their reading problems, often offering advice as much as asking for it. The teacher establishes the framework and the atmosphere of the lesson and provides suitable resources and guidance where necessary. Mutual stimulation, self-analysis and independent learning are the factors which make this approach different.

Discussion of favourite books raises the children's interest and desire to become more fluent in reading. Motivation increases as skills improve. At the end of a comparatively short period (three months maximum) of intensive involvement in the REG scores relating to both accuracy and comprehension improve, often dramatically. Subsequent monitoring of these children reveals that the benefits of the REG are sustained after they have returned to the normal remedial regime.

MATHEMATICS EXTENSION GROUP (MEG)

The success of the reading project in building pupils' confidence led to the development of a parallel scheme for children with intransigent numeracy problems. These lessons also involve the children in taking more responsibility for identifying their preferred learning strategies and for analysing the difficulties presented by particular areas of mathematics. The children exchange helpful tips with each other. They learn the benefits of risk taking within the safe confines of a group where privacy is respected. The other members provide encouragement and the teacher endorses the discovery method, praises and admires and avoids playing an authoritative role.

SOCIAL SKILLS

Poor social skills damage a child's self-esteem and can distract from the task in hand. For certain children timetabled remedial input in this specific area can be of great benefit. Groups of children meet weekly for an hour-long social session, usually under the supervision of the

Occupational Therapist and the Speech Therapist and sometimes with the involvement of a remedial teacher.

The children are selected through consultation between members of the remedial team and classteachers. The Educational Psychologist or Headteacher may also make specific recommendations. The pupils chosen are those who have particular difficulty relating to their peers and who are often inappropriate in their social responses. The group might include the child with particularly poor listening skills, one who taunts and provokes or another who is painfully shy and unassertive.

By videoing individual reactions, self-analysis is encouraged. Games, role play and problem-solving exercises help to develop easier social interaction. Although their problems are diverse, the children become mutually supportive and there is cohesion within the groups. At the end of a term of such sessions classteachers and parents report that all the children seem more relaxed and self-aware in their social interactions.

ART THERAPY

Art therapy is a further extension of the remedial programme. These sessions enable children to share with others creative experiences in a variety of media. It has proved a successful experiment with children who are poor risk-takers and particularly with those who are under-confident. The usual criteria of 'right' and 'wrong' do not apply when the activity involves the exploration of the possibilities inherent in a wide range of art materials. Sessions are held with a trained Art Therapist. The principles of privacy and confidentiality are respected. No visitors are allowed. Products can be taken home or to the classroom or torn up and destroyed, at the individual child's discretion. Free choice in 'Art Share' gives them a sense of being in control. It is safe to experiment. At regular intervals the Art Therapist instigates a discussion whereby the children can vent feelings of frustration, anger or humiliation. They can profitably counsel each other and increase their own self-respect as they are offered encouragement, sympathy, advice and support from the therapist and from others in the group.

Broadening the base of remediation

A delicate balance must be achieved between activities which enhance self-esteem, foster social skills and increase confidence and the commitment to deliver an intensive programme which teaches the basic academic skills and a full curriculum of subjects.

A typical example is the school play. A huge outlay of time and energy is necessary to achieve a stage production which impresses parents and which provides a memorable experience for the children. It can be argued that participation in a first-class performance is the experience of a lifetime. The very dyslexic children who would certainly have been passed over in mainstream school as being incompetent to read, let alone learn their parts, reveal hidden talents as they develop their roles with originality and panache. On the other hand a full-scale dramatic production can disrupt the timetable for weeks, with lessons and remedial sessions cancelled and with the disadvantages of the physical chaos created by scenery, costumes and props. However, the improvement of the children's self-image may need to be placed higher on the agenda than the strict observation of the school schedule and annual plays accepted as a valuable learning experience. At least it can be argued that the reading of parts, the memorizing of lines and the sequencing of scenes are all promoting useful skills. The remedial teachers can help the individual children to acquire them.

Similarly, outside visits, the week-long field trips, matches and concerts upset the timetable and can disturb vulnerable children, who dislike departure from normal routines. Travel, and particularly nights spent away from home, can create high stress levels. One advantage of engaging in these various activities is to help the more timid pupils to cope with this stress, particularly when they discover that such experiences can be thoroughly enjoyable. Another is that it gives the school a more 'normal' image and this is important if the children are to realize that they attend a 'specialist' rather than a 'special' school and can be proud that they have been selected to be pupils there.

Conclusion

Of all the professionals working at Fairley House, the remedial teachers play a role within the school which is probably least typical of universal practice. At the worst end of the spectrum remedial teachers in some schools still work 'in the broom cupboard'. They are quite likely to be part-time and sometimes do not even participate in staff meetings or attend parents' evenings. They tend to be somewhat marginalized within the framework of their school and have little influence in establishing policy or influencing procedures. Yet the full integration of the work of the remedial teacher with that undertaken in the classroom makes it possible to capitalize on their particular expertise and insight. This can lead to teaching methods being modified and different learning styles being identified. Crossfertilization takes place and everyone benefits. The remedial teachers are often the catalysts. They are therefore a crucial element in the professional team which is breaking down the barriers to learning which confront the individual child.

References

Augur, J. and Briggs, S. (1992) *The Hickey Multisensory Language Course*, Whurr, London.

Barkley, R. (1990) *Attention Deficit Hyperactivity Disorder: A Handbook for Diagnosis and Treatment*, Guilford Press, New York.

Buzan, T. (1993) *The Mind Map Book – Radiant Thinking*, BBC Books, London.

Cohen, J. (1994) On the differential diagnosis of reading, attentional and depressive disorders. *Annals of Dyslexia, an Interdisciplinary Journal of the Orton Dyslexia Society*, **XLIV**, 165–84.

Cooke, A. (1993) *Tackling Dyslexia the Bangor Way*, Whurr, London.

Hardman, F. and Beverton, S. (1993) Cooperative group work and the development of metadiscoursal skills. *Serving Special Educational Needs*, 8(4), 146–50.

Hornsby, B. and Shear, F. (1994) *Alpha to Omega. The A–Z of Teaching Reading, Writing and Spelling*, 4th edn, Heinemann Educational Books, London.

Lebeer, J. (1995) Conductive education and the mediated learning experience theory of Feuerstein. *European Journal of Special Needs Education*, **10**(2), 124–37.

Miles, E. (1992) *The Bangor Dyslexia Teaching System*, 2nd edn, Whurr, London.

Wechsler, D. (1991) *The Wechsler Intelligence Scale for Children*, 3rd edn, NFER, Slough.

9 The class teacher

Angela Dominy and Nicholas Rees

The chapter by Nick Rees and Angela Dominy on the work of the class teacher follows ideally after Patience Thomson's description of the work of the remedial teacher in an individual and small group context. The impact on specific learning disabilities is so much more effective when class teachers are aware of the precise nature of a child's difficulties and how they can help and support the work of the specialists around them. Liaison and teamwork are the keys to success. Nick and Angela have worked for many years with children with a variety of symptoms associated with specific learning disabilities and bring to their chapter this wealth of experience.

Introduction

The following passage, written by James, an 11-year-old dyslexic boy, recording a recent visit to the Royal Institution for a lecture, is remarkable in several ways. The boy in question had written no notes. He was relying on memory. He had obviously taken an intelligent interest and had understood what was going on. Yet his written language has a bizarre quality with words so ill spelt that his text is almost impossible to interpret. For the child this is embarrassing, for the teacher frustrating. Above all, it is perplexing. Such work is typical of the dyslexic.

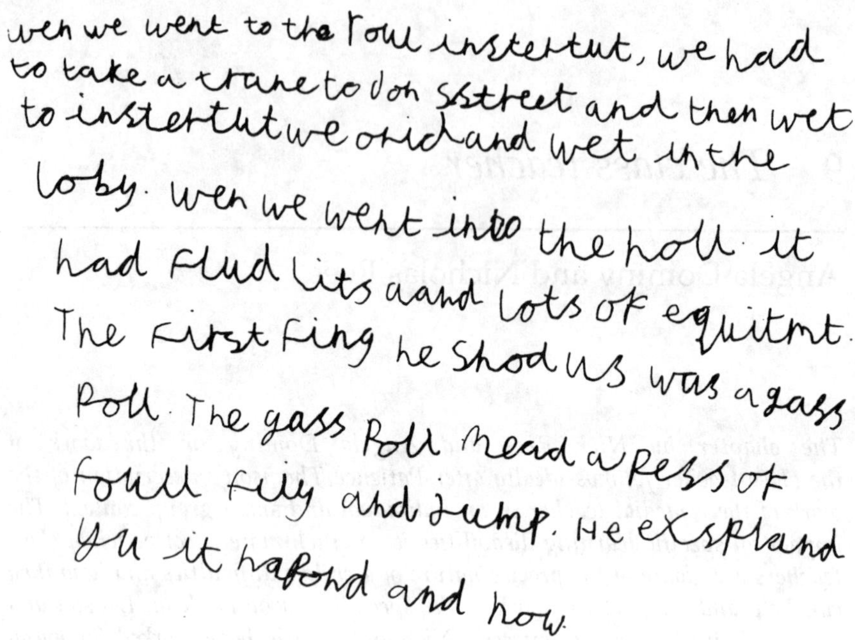

wen we went to the roul instertut, we had to take a trane to don ssstreet and then wet to instertut we onid and wet in the loby. wen we went into the holl. it had flud lits aand lots of equitmt. The first fing he shod us was a gass poll. The gass poll mead a ress of foull fiiy and jump. He exspland yu it hafond and how.

Fig. 9.1

When we went to the Royal Institution, we had to take a train to Bond Street and then went to the Institution. We arrived and went into the lobby. Then we went into the hall. It had flood lights and lots of equipment. The first thing he showed us was a glass pole. The glass pole made a piece of foil fly and jump. He explained why it happened and how.

This passage continued for a further 12 lines making it quite clear that James had fully understood the content of the lecture despite the considerable dyslexic evidence in his written expression.

Educational profiles

In order to understand how dyslexic children function in the classroom, it is necessary to compare their psychological profile and academic performance with those of children who have no dyslexic symptoms. The latter exhibit a more generally consistent profile and their educational development is more logical and predictable. If they show competence in acquiring proficient literacy skills, they will normally do well in most academic subjects. If they are 'slow learners', they will experience difficulties in every area. When performance does not match potential, there are often obvious external factors which have affected the non-dyslexic child's academic progress, such as prolonged school absences, poor teaching or emotional or psychological problems. In contrast, though dyslexic children are naturally not immune to the influences of external factors, the ever-widening gap between their potential and their poor performance can appear mystifying, until a careful diagnosis of their specific learning difficulties has been made and the nature of these difficulties determined.

DYSLEXIC PROFILES

Not all dyslexic pupils present the same profile. Each individual displays a different pattern of strengths and weaknesses. However, in the classroom certain characteristics are often evident which may either be the result or the cause of their problems. By the time they are in their second or third year of school they are often suffering from low self-esteem, having already failed academically in several areas but most noticeably in the acquisition of basic literacy and numeracy skills. They may also have failed socially as well. They lack confidence and this can manifest itself in many ways, including attention-seeking behaviour, withdrawal, aggression or a generally antisocial, anti-authoritarian attitude.

The dyslexic child can feel victimized. They may well have been made to feel stupid and are aware of the constant veiled criticism that they are unintelligent, unmotivated or careless, that they have only 'to try harder' to succeed. The teacher who, to be sympathetic and supportive, gives them less demanding tasks and seemingly unwarranted praise may well appear patronizing. The child reacts by becoming unhappy and may well show visible signs of stress. At home there may be temper tantrums, bedwetting or even, in extreme cases, school phobia. At school there may be evidence of non-co-operation, diversionary tactics, aggression, misbehaviour and withdrawal. In severe cases of stress the child may require the advice and help of a doctor, psychotherapist or other professional. The common factors which may cause stress include a lack of confidence, low self-esteem, failure, insecurity, vulnerability, lack of control, teasing, lack of understanding and support from parents, teachers and peers.

INCONSISTENT PERFORMANCE

The dyslexic child's performance is likely to be inconsistent, with discrepancies between different curriculum areas. Although a child may excel in grasping mathematics or scientific concepts, their literacy skills may be very weak. A child who has mastered reading may have severe difficulties with spelling or comprehension, with organization skills or with maths. Dyslexic children do not have global problems, but disconcerting gaps in their knowledge related to their strengths and weaknesses. They will, however, predictably experience learning difficulties throughout the school day from their time of arrival to the time of departure. The less informed help they receive and the less chance they are given to succeed, the greater will be the level of stress engendered by a typical school day.

LANGUAGE PROCESSING

Most dyslexic children experience difficulties with language processing, which may well include oral communication and particularly written work. These are skills which are constantly required in academic work. Because of the extra effort involved, these children may have a comparatively short attention span and tire easily. Many exhibit a lack of confidence and are unsure of themselves, even when their understanding and application are sound. Dyslexic children use evasion strategies, distracting attention from the task with acts of bravado, daydreaming, joking or claiming to feel unwell. Such strategies are only of limited efficacy and may well invite adult disapproval and negative reactions, which can only increase the stress levels of the child.

ORAL COMMUNICATION

Though often apparently articulate, the dyslexic child may well have problems with oral communication. With regard to spoken language, there can be difficulties with the pronunciation of words, which may become muddled, with syllables transposed, omitted or added. The dyslexic child may have word-finding or naming difficulties when trying to explain something. Poor expressive skills are often in evidence, though they may have a good vocabulary. The structure of language may be poorly understood or expressed. There are often comprehension difficulties, a result of poor information processing, particularly if instructions are complicated or multiple. A few dyslexics have articulation problems. Such possible areas of weakness hamper competent and effective communication not only with the teachers but with classroom peers, creating tension and misunderstandings.

READING

Dyslexic children may have difficulty mastering the first stage of reading because of inherent difficulties in learning the letters of the alphabet. Regardless of age, the non-reader has to acquire and apply knowledge of sound–symbol relationships before progress can be made. Pupils may read slowly word by word without meaning, reverse letters, omit word endings or whole words, substitute words or transpose letters or syllables. Others may line slip or lose their place completely.

WRITTEN WORK

The cause of dyslexic children's problems is not necessarily the same in every case. For instance, many dyslexic children are slow to produce written work, but there may be different reasons for their inhibitions. Some exhibit fine motor difficulties and without help and continued guidance may continue to have a poor pencil grip, poor formation of letters and little knowledge of joined handwriting. Since writing is physically laborious, little is achieved. They may have poor visual sequencing and/or poor visual memory for signs and symbols and experience difficulties in writing letters and words in the correct order. They may be inefficient at copying written work far-point (from the board) or near-point (from a text book). They may produce letter reversals, rotations and transpositions when writing and spelling. A prime cause of their failure to do justice to themselves in their written work is their justified lack of confidence in their spelling, which at best is inaccurate and at worst bizarre or even totally incomprehensible. The planning, organization, presentation and execution of written work can all present separate problems for the dyslexic child.

ORGANIZATION

From a practical point of view, dyslexic children are often poorly organized. They find it difficult to be at the right place, with the correct items, at the specified time. Their desks and school bags are usually messy. They have difficulties with the sequencing of time and may be unaware of the time of day. They are often slow to learn to read a watch or clock. They may think it is lunch time when it is only mid-morning or already time to go home. They have little awareness of the significance of dates, not knowing how long it is until the end of term, their birthday or Christmas. Their behaviour can be inconsequential in relation to time and they can appear lost and confused. They cannot judge how long a piece of work will take them or plan their time sensibly.

MANUAL DEXTERITY

Dyslexic children may suffer from poor manual dexterity and be clumsy. They may have a poor sense of direction and be confused by such concepts as left and right, before and after, under and over, second and third or longer and longest. This has often been a reason for getting into a lot of trouble in mainstream school, when motives have been mis-interpreted. They are not necessarily disobedient or destructive, but could merely be confused and clumsy.

PROBLEMS WITH HOMEWORK

Dyslexic pupils frequently experience problems with homework. They find it difficult to settle down of their own accord and need to be taught a set routine. They may confuse or miss out part of verbal instructions. Written instructions may have been copied incorrectly or incompletely. In mainstream school they may experience stress because the work takes them far longer than would normally be expected. Dyslexic children are easily distracted and are unduly affected by any factors at home which make it difficult for them to work quietly and independently. It should also be noted that they are often significantly more tired than the average child at the end of the school day, since they have had to put more effort into every aspect of their work.

SOCIAL SKILLS

A lack of social skills resulting from poor self-esteem can affect these children's lives in almost every way. Many have experienced earlier rejection by their peer group in a previous school and know failure very well. They may behave and communicate inappropriately with both teachers and peer group. They may not know how to involve themselves in group situations or display such antisocial behaviour that they are excluded by their peer group. Lateness, disorganization, clumsiness and an unkempt appearance all contribute towards a lack of acceptance.

ACCENTUATING THE POSITIVE

Dyslexic children may be unable to show or reveal their strengths. Everybody has strengths, but dyslexic children are often unable to draw on theirs in a positive way. Many of these strengths are practical in nature, in areas such as design, art, computers and sport. Others have an excellent general knowledge and can verbalize their many thoughts and ideas. It might seem surprising that a lack of literacy skills should inhibit their creativity but usually it does because, for example, they cannot read instructions. This leads to frustration.

WITHDRAWAL FROM MAINSTREAM EDUCATION

The decision to take dyslexic children out of the mainstream classroom and transfer them for a period to an environment of total immersion in a remedial programme is not one which is taken lightly. There must be a degree of confidence that a child could not successfully remain in mainstream school even if some remedial support were available and that the prognosis for progress in a specialist environment is acceptable positive, with provision that will be appropriate and adequate.

Assessment procedures – class teacher

The class teacher has a role to play in the initial assessment of the child. Possible candidates may be brought into the classroom for the day if there is any doubt about their academic, emotional or behavioural capacity to cope. The teacher can then help to assess their suitability for full-time integration into a programme of total immersion. Of particular concern will be the child's ability to interact effectively with their peer group in the various classes, during lunch and break times, to respond to the structure of the class and to the teacher and to keep up with the academic demands of the curriculum. It can also be very useful for a classteacher to have had firsthand experience of how well a child is functioning and at what level of skills and maturity, so that they can be correctly placed in a suitable class on entry to the school. This is valuable where there is a particularly wide gap between a child's chronological age and their reading and spelling ability, as placement in these cases can be difficult. You cannot, for example, incorporate a 10-year-old with non-existent reading skills into a reception class of 6- and 7-year-old non-starters.

INFORMATION FROM PROFESSIONAL ASSESSMENTS

Class teachers refer to the tests carried out by the Educational Psychologist and other professionals at assessment to extract information regarding children's strengths and weaknesses and draw implications for teaching style and content. Multidisciplinary assessments will have screened out children who have educational difficulties but who are not dyslexic, such as those who have English as a foreign language, are of low ability, have behaviour or emotional problems, are hyperactive or who have been poorly taught or missed a lot of school.

There are a number of different conclusions which can be drawn from the professional reports. If they show evidence of poor auditory recall, then the child will have problems in class with responding to verbal instructions.

Children who have a high average score in the visual subtests are more likely to make progress when the material is presented through the visual channel. Alternatively a pupil with poor visual skills will not cope if given a large amount of far-point copying from the board. Those pupils with poor fine motor control will have great difficulty with handwriting and the presentation of their work.

The task of the class teacher is to unlock the pupil's potential using all the information available to determine how the pupil will learn most effectively. Class teachers can relate back to the original reports when difficulties emerge and establish realistic goals. Family questionnaires, which may include compounding factors such as a death in the family or sibling rivalry, may give more relevance to the teacher's understanding of the pupil's inability to make progress.

Incorporating the remedial programme into the classroom

Integrating remediation with classwork is not uncommon in mainstream schools and is sometimes achieved through providing a support teacher within the classroom. At Fairley House the specialist remedial teachers, Speech Therapists and Occupational Therapists also work within the classroom on a daily basis to ensure an integrated approach, while also working individually with the pupils on a withdrawal system. The aim is to deliver both the National Curriculum and a full remedial programme, modifying and adapting the approach to take account of the pupil's specific learning difficulties.

The remedial approach is sustained throughout the school day and incorporates team teaching methods with individual and group lessons. Every member of the team gains through this approach by viewing the child holistically. There are frequent opportunities for direct communication between staff and for closer observation of the pupils. Greater insight for designing and reviewing a child's individual needs is provided. Planning begins at the assessment stage. Subsequent records compiled by all relevant in-house professionals are used to help build up the child's individual education plan and determine the most effective teaching methods. Emphasis can be laid on the pupil's strengths, which can be channelled into strategies to reduce problems.

THE CURRICULUM

The curriculum subjects are covered in group situations by class teachers and reinforced by specialist remedial staff. The school day is based on a structured, logical timetable, which enables the child to become familiar with a regular daily routine. In the first part of the morning, every child attends lessons in reading, spelling, handwriting and mathematics. There are great advantages if these more structured lessons take place in the morning, when the pupils are fresh and able to concentrate for longer periods. The children can be grouped according to their ability, the nature of their specific problems and their physical and emotional maturity, in order for them to receive the exact level and type of tuition they require. As the whole school studies these subjects at the same time, there is flexibility within the time-table for children to change ability groups as and when necessary. Matching of skill levels must not be the only criterion; age and maturity should also always be considered. The sharing of responsibility in deciding placement means that the pupils receive more appropriate individual help and it also creates a more targeted system. Such co-operation, beginning at the planning stage, enables the professionals involved to have a broader knowledge of the children they teach and there is a closer analysis of children's progress due to discussion within the team.

THE NATIONAL CURRICULUM

Pupils follow the National Curriculum, details of which can be found in a number of directives published by the Department for Education and Employment. English, science and mathematics are classified as 'core' subjects. Other subjects taught include design technology, information technology, geography, history, art, music, physical educa-tion, drama and religious education. All subjects are modified where necessary to make them more accessible to the pupils. A small group of older pupils may have access to French on an oral basis, which intro-duces them to a modern foreign language before transferring to secondary education.

The aim is to allow pupils access to a broad and balanced curriculum, to develop their learning and experience and to prepare them to return to conventional education. Such access may have been denied them in the past in a mainstream school environment, because the teaching methods were not appropriate for dyslexic children with inadequate learning skills.

TEACHING MODIFICATIONS

The teacher needs to take all the specific difficulties of the dyslexic child into consideration when planning lessons. Since the pattern of difficulty of the individual child may vary considerably, flexibility will be essential. The main challenge is the need to combine remedia-tion with the delivery of a full curriculum. Modifications are usually applied both in the use of differentiated material and in the way the curriculum is presented to the pupils. A different teaching style is required. Small classes are also important if the responses of individual children are to be closely monitored.

MULTISENSORY APPROACHES

It is important to engage all the dyslexic child's pathways to learning by using a multisensory approach in all activities. By associating the visual, auditory and kinaesthetic modalities simultaneously, the child will learn most effectively by seeing, hearing and doing. Kinaesthetic learning is the perception obtained through muscle awareness and movement. For example, where a child is required to learn about scale they will do so most successfully if they can see what scale is, listen to an explanation of what scale means and have 'hands-on' experience making a scale model of their bedroom or classroom. Dyspraxic children may have problems with practical tasks and may need a lot of help and encouragement, using alternative strategies to meet success.

MOTIVATION THROUGH ENCOURAGEMENT

It is also important to accentuate the strengths and talents of pupils, to encourage each child to be positive and confident of their ultimate success and to maintain interest and motivation. Weaknesses need to be minimized and failure should be avoided whenever possible. It can be helpful for the teacher to break tasks down into small identifiable units, so that pupils experience a degree of success at each stage of the task before tackling the next. The teacher should ensure that the child has mastered both methods and concepts at each level before proceeding further.

INFORMATION PROCESSING

Since dyslexic children so often have problems with absorbing information through the auditory channel and have a short attention span, teaching styles need to be adapted, limiting the amount of verbal information given at any one time. Teachers should speak clearly and slowly to allow time for effective language processing. It is often necessary for the teacher to question the pupils to check that they have understood. It is a useful exercise for the child to put the instruction or explanation into their own words. Visual reinforcement in the form of chronological time lines, calendars, graphs and lists of relevant vocabulary are particularly important in the teaching of dyslexic children, who will refer to them more than usual. They should be in bold print and simply presented.

Essential aids should be utilized in as many ways as possible around the classroom, on the wall, on the child's desk and in their books. They give support to pupils with poor recall ability for names and specific words. Concrete aids such as counters, blocks and models of mathematical shapes, plastic or wooden letters or geographical 3D models are helpful to the dyslexic pupil, who finds it difficult to decode or remember the written symbol or word.

Children are generally able to discuss and converse in an intelligent manner, but the teacher must reduce the level of expectation for written work, which often does not reflect intellectual ability. Written work should not be marked on spelling but on content. Specific strategies should be taught to facilitate personal organization and presentation, so that all work is properly planned and executed. Consistency is important.

TIME FACTORS

When planning the timetable and curriculum content for dyslexic children, it must be remembered that more time may be necessary to cover the work, since it is often delivered in smaller modules and consolidation is essential. More oral discussion needs to take place than in mainstream teaching and material may have to be presented in more than one way. Texts may need to be abridged or the print enlarged or interpreted. Pupils may need to have a copy of the texts or instructions in front of them while the teacher reads them aloud to ensure an accurate interpretation of the content. Work may need to be colour coded or numbered in sequence. It may be advisable to present only one aspect of the material at a time to prevent overload. Work will take a more practical approach with pupils getting 'hands-on' experience as they talk through or read about a topic. The use of auditory, visual and tactile aids is encouraged in all subjects. Helpful guidelines and key words to explain the concept would be displayed as further visual reinforcement.

COPYING TASKS

Much of the work is organized without having to copy from books or from the board, since many dyslexic pupils are slow and inaccurate at doing this. Pictorial representations are used whenever possible instead of standard texts. When writing on a chalk or whiteboard different coloured markers can be used for each line to prevent a pupil line slipping during a task requiring copying.

INDIVIDUAL TUITION

Specific remedial teaching for the individual child is covered on a one-to-one or small group basis by Speech and Language Therapists, Occupational Therapists and other qualified remedial teachers. Children follow individual programmes based on their personal range of strengths and weaknesses in the areas of handwriting, gross and fine motor skills, visual–perceptual skills, auditory skills, oral language, comprehension, creative writing and in maths. The remedial staff, in close liaison with the class teacher, can determine the areas where children need targeted individual support or more intensively concentrated tuition. They can also focus on the child's individual need for instruction in specific areas.

Teaching reading skills

There are many facets to reading and the decoding of text with accuracy and fluency is only one aspect of a complex skill. Comprehension is equally important. Initially children may need to follow a graded reading scheme, but the long-term aim must be to introduce them to a wide range of material, fiction and non-fiction, and to help them to make best use of it. Eventually they must learn to interpret, predict, evaluate and summarize.

To this end, the dyslexic child needs an intensive programme. Daily small group reading sessions should be established, within which the children should be well matched in ability. Additional regular class-room practice is important in developing reading skills. Skills such as being able to take turns, following and keeping their place in the text, improving fluency and accuracy, discussing the use and meaning of punctuation and paragraphs, selecting appropriate books, mastering sustained reading, skimming and scanning for specific purposes and using a library and understanding its organization may need a lot of practice before acquisition. Variety is important and tapes, games and group discussions can all be incorporated. Computer programs can also support the development of reading.

PARENTS' INPUT

Parental support at home is also a major factor and should include providing a quiet place in which to read and a selection of suitable reading material. Children who are not competent readers may well benefit from paired or shared reading when parent and child read together, with parents discontinuing their contribution whenever the child feels confident to continue alone. Whereas for ordinary children this is help-ful, for dyslexic children it is essential.

MATERIALS

The frustrations associated with reading failure escalate dramatically as the child grows older and the demands within the conventional class-room increase. For example, once a child reaches the age of nine or ten, competent reading skills are a prerequisite for coping with the main-stream curriculum. They are also needed for general survival in school, for reading notices on the board, timetables and instructions. As the child progresses through school, the shortfall in basic reading skills becomes increasingly apparent to the teacher, to the peer group and, very importantly, to the child themselves. Parents and teachers may put increasing pressure on the child as they see the gap widening.

Children who have a reading age significantly lower than their chronological age often become frustrated with the material they have to read. Reading material must be pitched at the right level for the child. It is demoralizing to struggle with a text or be bored. High interest level is vital for good motivation for reading, which must be maintained if reading skills are to be improved. It is very important for children with reading difficulties to progress slowly and lay sound foundations in order to build up secure reading and comprehension skills before attempting books which are more challenging. The teacher has the diffi-cult job of directing the child so that they remain interested and achieve a high success rate. A reasonable print size is also an important factor as this makes it easier to follow the text without line slipping, losing the place or muddling the words. Care must be taken in all these areas of reading to ensure that it is not the discouraging, demoralizing and humiliating experience which it may have been in the past. Reading must be promoted as enjoyable, relaxing and informative but above all fun.

Teaching spelling skills

Written language is a very difficult area for most dyslexic children to master. They may have weak information processing, inadequate expressive and receptive language skills and problems with both spelling and handwriting. These areas can be taught and remediated separately, but it is important to show how they interact, otherwise the children are unable to use their skills flexibly and efficiently.

An effective programme should be highly structured, multisensory and cumulative, i.e. logical and consistent. Ideally it should use a system which teaches reading, writing and spelling by engaging the visual, auditory and kinaesthetic or tactile channels simultaneously. Dyslexic pupils do not generally learn to read and spell by a process of 'Look and Say' or 'Look and Remember'. They have to be taught how words are constructed both visually and auditorily. Where other children easily pick up concepts of rhyme and pattern, dyslexic pupils must be taught to do this slowly and carefully. Linkages between the auditory and visual and sensory channels help to reinforce concepts.

A MULTISENSORY APPROACH

It is helpful for these children to spell by analogy. This method works on the belief that if a child can spell 'fat', then they can also spell 'hat', 'mat', 'cat' and 'sat' because they are orthographically similar. The visual pattern reinforces the phonic pattern. It makes sense to group words into families. This is the easiest way for the child to build up a knowledge of regular orthographic and phonic patterns. Priority is given to the major patterns and one should then move on to the lesser used patterns and exceptions.

Children learn letter names and letter sounds and how to recognize letter shapes. It is very important for dyslexic children to hear a sound, see it presented visually or, in the early stages, kinaesthetically with plastic or wooden letters and to produce the symbol with a finger, a pencil or whole arm through 'skywriting'. This method strengthens the child's awareness of what written language is all about and most importantly, enables them to begin to link sounds to their corresponding symbols. It is important to insist that sounds and symbols are always linked.

Spelling can successfully be taught in small carefully matched groups on a daily basis. Each session should be structured to include different activities which make use of the different sensory channels for the most effective learning.

Spelling lessons contain certain typical elements. The alphabet is taught through various activities. The children can use plastic or wooden 3D letters and arrange the alphabet in its proper sequence. They can practise techniques such as sequencing, concepts of 'before' and 'after' and prepare for dictionary work. Cards can be displayed for the children to identify and name each letter, digraph or blend and to translate them into speech sounds.

When being introduced to a new sound for spelling, the children learn through the discovery method by hearing it, seeing the letters which spell it and touching an object related to the new sound. The final part of discovery is tactile. The child is presented with a 'feelie' bag, a fabric bag containing a hidden object with the sound and spelling 'or' in its name, for example a fork. Each child feels in the bag without looking to discover the object just by touch. The object will then become the key word for future phonic work. These new sounds are then introduced for reading, writing and spelling.

Spelling practice supports the pupil's application of sound-symbol relationships learned through the spelling cards. One method used at Fairley House, based on phonic principles, is simultaneous oral spelling (Cox, 1977) and otherwise known to the children as 'Save Our Spelling' (SOS). The routine is used as follows.

- The teacher says the word clearly.
- The child listens and watches.
- The child repeats the word.
- The child sounds out the letters.
- The child names the letters aloud.
- The child writes the letters simultaneously naming them again.
- The child checks the spelling, reading the whole word.

A brief review of the work covered that day encourages pupils by showing them specifically what they have learned. They too must appreciate that the programme is not only cumulative but finite.

A typical lesson could involve any of the following tasks.

- A review of learned letter patterns using a letter pack with key word pictures.
- Introducing the sound and the letters by a look, listen and echo sequence.
- Practising the letter pattern.
- Discovering the key word.
- Reading the words for meaning.
- Matching the order of the sound to its position in a word.
- Finding other words to fit the pattern.
- Rhyming, dictation, free writing, word searches, quizzes and crosswords.

The key element of learning these patterns and rules is to increase the pupils' ability to transfer these literacy skills into their writing.

Children can also be taught the segmentation of words for both reading and spelling. They are encouraged to listen and look for smaller words or parts of a word within a longer multisyllable word. If a child can read and spell 'count', then the word 'encounter' is less of a challenge. For this method to be truly effective, the child needs to be aware of syllable division within a word, as well as practising visual retention of letter clusters. They must understand syllabic units and phonemic units within a word. It may be necessary to work for some time on syllable division before it becomes an automatic response. For this purpose children can be taught to tap or clap out the syllables they hear in a word, for example, re/mem/ber.

Sight words are also part of this structured programme. A sight word is any word that cannot be sounded out phonetically and therefore needs to be learned separately because it does not belong to a word family. 'Said' and 'because' are good examples. Priority is given to common words and those relevant to the pupil's experience, for example, words associated with the term's topic. Words which have a rule, but with only a few examples relevant to the child's vocabulary, such as 'steak', 'break' and 'great', are also included as sight words.

One successful method for learning sight words is the Fernald tracing technique (Fernald, 1943). The pupil reads the word aloud and then traces over the whole word with the index finger, naming each letter as they write and repeats this process three times before writing the word again without visual clues. This method of learning irregular words has a very good success rate because it incorporates the visual, auditory and kinaesthetic modes of learning simultaneously.

TEACHING BASIC SKILLS TO OLDER CHILDREN

Older primary-age children who are still having problems acquiring basic literacy skills will need a more sophisticated approach. Suffixes and prefixes can be introduced as early as possible in the programme and syllable division needs to be taught as an important skill, as it increases word attack skills and the general confidence of the children. Many longer words are, in fact, more logical in their spelling patterns.

Children with continuing spelling problems at the age of nine and beyond need this type of stimulus. Some of these older children may have some knowledge of phonic rules, but it is patchy and insecure. Initial testing will discover how much they know already and foundations can be consolidated. A great deal of time can be saved if the teaching effort is concentrated on what the child does not know, rather than rigorously allotting time to all spelling patterns and rules regardless of the child's previous knowledge and experience. It cannot be stressed enough that spelling needs to be fun and to be made interesting and pupils need to know that the major spelling patterns and rules cover the majority of words in the English language.

Pupils who have experienced a great deal of failure and feel stressed during tests can have spelling 'checks' instead, which can be done orally with the teacher writing the words down or done in a fun way with the pupil hopping on a 'rocker' board or bouncing on a trampoline during their turn while they call out the spellings. Pupils are involved in a multisensory way, writing on the board and making games as well as transferring their increased spelling knowledge to their writing. The children are encouraged to incorporate in their stories words taken from spelling families which they have learned previously.

Teaching more advanced literacy skills

WRITTEN WORK

Non-dyslexic children may discuss a subject in class with their peers and teacher. When asked to record what they have learned on paper, they will be able to produce written facts which reflect their intellectual grasp of the content of the earlier discussion. When children are asked to write, they need to be competent in both advanced aspects of literacy and in communication skills. They need to conceptualize, sequence their thoughts, use syntax, spelling, grammar, punctuation and handwriting. They must plan not only the content but also the presentation of their work. All this makes the act of writing extremely demanding and it is not surprising to observe in dyslexic children's writing that although, with training, they may be reasonably competent in all of these areas in isolation, the effort involved when it is necessary to use all these skills at the same time results in a breakdown of quality.

Some dyslexic children may be able to sustain a high level of oral discussion. When it comes to recording this on paper, the teacher has to make allowances for the child's disabilities with the written word. Many need to talk around the subject, collecting ideas from each other and making their own ideas clearer in their minds. This will often take a long time to get started. Some will give up at the beginning, before committing pen to paper, as failure is so deep rooted. Without careful plans in note form and spelling lists which include key words, many pupils will write very little.

Younger children may need to be encouraged with a storyboard displaying a sequence of pictures. Some may not be able to come up with any ideas for titles and a range of these are useful to have on hand. It is necessary to build up their writing, sentence by sentence, using planning skills. Many will also need extra time to complete the task. Some pupils can tire easily, as they are having to think about so many aspects of writing, and then want to bring the story to an abrupt end. Others write quickly and carelessly, forgetting every aspect of spelling, grammar, punctuation, presentation and handwriting, as they cannot focus on anything more than getting their ideas on the page.

POSITIVE FEEDBACK

It is often necessary for the teacher to encourage and persuade the child that writing is both a valuable and an essential skill, which can be enjoyable as well. The experienced teacher knows that written language skills will be more successfully developed and have more meaning through the purposeful use of written language related to a current topic or the child's own interest rather than through the use of random exercises divorced from context. Flair, imagination and insight are necessary if the dyslexic child is to be challenged and reassured.

FURTHER TEACHING TECHNIQUES

Children are encouraged to write in a variety of styles at their own pace, with the teacher teaching to the particular areas of weakness such as content, spelling or layout. Structured handwriting guidelines, pencil grips and posture all play an important part and many dyslexic pupils may need individual or small group handwriting sessions. The teacher must take into account what can be expected of the pupils at their current skill level. Pupils should be introduced to, and learn to master, a variety of writing skills and should be aware of their audience. They should be able to write creatively and with imagination to create coherent, sequenced stories. The ability to write with accuracy a list of instructions or details about a certain place, subject or experiment must be developed. They should write freely about personal experiences, including thoughts and feelings. They should learn to compose formal and informal letters, poetry (which need not necessarily rhyme), notes as an aid to learning or as a prompt for memory and plans for compositions. Touch typing, word processing, proofreading and editing are all skills which help the dyslexic pupil. Naturally all these skills cannot be taught simultaneously and current priorities must constantly be monitored.

As a writing activity senior children can write adventure stories for the junior pupils. This demands extensive communication between author and intended reader and can be a huge source of remediation in itself, instilling a sense of pride and purpose in the finished article.

Teaching mathematics

The importance of discussion and explanation in maths cannot be over-emphasized. This must not come from the teacher alone; the child should be a contributor. The vocabulary of mathematics overlaps with the more conventional use of English but there are discrepancies which need to be explained to the dyslexic child, whose processing of language is often more literal than that of their peers. The terms 'sum of' or the 'difference between' can be very confusing. Some may have problems with concepts of 'above' and 'below', 'higher' and 'lower', 'greater' and 'lesser', which lead to considerable difficulty in interpreting instructions or memorizing concepts.

LANGUAGE PROBLEMS

If children are experiencing difficulties with the language of mathematics, the Speech Therapist can often help in this area by working in one-to-one lessons on problem solving and interpreting questions in order that the children gain a working understanding of mathematical words. Many different words are used in maths to mean the same thing. For example:

- addition can be: sum of, increase, +, plus, and, total, more than, add, altogether, greater than or count on;
- subtraction can be: less than, decrease, –, subtract, take away, difference, minus, count back, reduce or short of;
- multiplication can be: multiply, times, ×, of, product or double.
- division can be: share, split, group into, how many, divide or ÷.

Even the visual signs are similar for addition (+) and multiplication (×), and subtraction (–) and equivalent (=).

PROBLEM SOLVING

Problem solving and investigation play an important role in mathematical learning and development. Dyslexic children need to know that they have the means to work through a problem and should be encouraged to use their own methods. Children must be taught to trust their own reasoning powers and explain their working. Mistakes should be recognized as a part of the natural learning process so that risk taking is encouraged, but eventual success must be recognized and reinforced. Some dyslexic pupils are good at mental arithmetic but are reluctant to put their workings and answers down on paper. This may be a problem due to poor sequencing or the result of poor fine motor skills or even a general lack of confidence and fear of failure. They often know the answer but do not know how they worked it out or cannot explain how they came about it. They have to be encouraged to record their workings on paper by being required to work through the stages slowly and methodically.

ACCELERATED LEARNING

In a large class the dyslexic pupil may wait too long before help is available and become discouraged or feel that not enough ground is being covered and become frustrated. If staff are teamed or paired for maths and children can be grouped according to skill level, then children are more likely to work at a similar pace and can receive more help and individual tuition. Pupils can change groups when appropriate.

There are some children who do not suffer from any difficulties in maths, despite their other learning disabilities, and these need the opportunity to work at a faster pace, with greater challenges.

FURTHER DIFFICULTIES

Poor information processing and problems with patterns and sequencing lead to a lack of internalization and understanding, which is often the main contributing factor to mathematical difficulties. Poor sequencing skills for symbols and concepts can be a great problem in the necessary stages of solving some mathematical problems. The teacher needs to work at a slow pace with the child, explaining, reinforcing and checking each stage with the pupils as they are taught.

It is good practice to require children to learn and repeat exactly the instructions for each stage of the sum. Dyslexic children tend to forget the type of sum and symbol they are working with. They often find it difficult to recall basic number facts such as number bonds and multiplication tables. It is important that children understand that they can solve problems without having instant recall of certain facts. They can use alternative strategies. It is possible to give the pupils table squares, 100 squares or teach them quick methods to calculate. More important, though, is teaching children to be methodical in their working, to make note of it and to check their answers.

For children who cannot read fluently, written mathematical questions present as a major problem before the mechanics can even be contemplated. They should be encouraged to read a sum in its entirety before working out the answer and at the end ask themselves: 'Does this make sense?' It may be helpful to teach them to rephrase the question to make sure that they have established the meaning.

SPATIAL PROBLEMS

Children with poor spatial awareness have problems with organizing their number work on a page. This may well lead to errors and confusion, even though the child may mentally be quite adept with numerical problems. Working on squared paper can help a great deal if children are taught to use one square for each digit. They also need to learn the importance of spacing and how to work in columns. Occupational Therapists can be helpfully involved with these specific difficulties. An inability to coordinate the size of the digits is not uncommon. Dyspraxic pupils may need even more help and guidance with 'rolling' rulers, using card not paper and by using larger squared graph paper.

Many children experience directional difficulties and are confused that they have learned to read and write from left to right but most sums are worked from right to left. Other directional problems are experienced with co-ordinates and points of the compass.

CONCRETE AIDS

Pupils should not be presented with the abstract concepts before they have fully understood the concrete implications. Dyslexic pupils tend to interpret what they learn too specifically and are less able to transfer their skills. They often compartmentalize and need specific exercises to teach them how to apply the theory in other situations. It is essential for all children to work with equipment such as beads, unifix cubes and coloured rods in order to gain a visual, tactile and mental experience of a numerical concept before they work with abstract problems. Dyslexic pupils have particular difficulty with written symbols and need to make use of concrete materials for much longer than might be expected. Learning can take place in a non-threatening way through the use of games and concrete materials and even through stories which feature mathematical elements.

CALCULATORS

Calculators are now an established item of classroom equipment, but can be particularly valuable to the dyslexic pupil who confuses mathematical signs. They provide a kinaesthetic approach and reinforce the difference between symbols by their position on the calculator keyboard. Calculators offer a visual way for pupils to check their own work. The visual input of the signs and numbers can reinforce a child's understanding of mathematics, while removing the possibility of making errors when calculating with pen and paper. Calculators can motivate and increase children's confidence in their mathematical ability.

COMPUTERS

The computer can be a great aid to dyslexic pupils in the area of maths because it is an effective visual aid and an immediate incentive for a reluctant mathematician. It often improves concentration. A number of computer programs offer the opportunity to explore shape and direction, number relationships and patterns, use of mental arithmetic, estimation, angles, distance, symmetry, enlargement and scale.

A database can be used to store and process information which has been collected as part of a survey. Graphs, charts and tables can all be produced to provide visual displays to interpret data. Word processors can be used to write stories involving mathematics. Teamwork amongst pupils is very important. For example, to practise recording data in maths, a weather station can be used and daily records kept for half a term. The information can then be put onto a database and graphs produced and interpreted.

Topic work

Science, geography and history are covered under various topic headings and are related to other areas of the curriculum. A 2-year plan has been developed with six topics: 'Ourselves', 'Air and Space', 'Growth', 'Energy and Forces', 'Communications' and 'Homes and Habitats'. Each topic lasts for a term. All the classes in the school cover the same topic, but at different levels of sophistication which allows for a considerable degree of cross-fertilization. It is often easier to link the scientific, geographical and historical aspects of a particular subject within the same lesson or series of lessons and within a limited time span. This way dyslexic children become totally involved in what they are doing. The specific topic-related vocabulary can be revised and checked and any misinterpretations discussed.

As the topic is organized within a whole-school approach, displays throughout the school are reinforcing the themes in pictorial or written form. Experiments in the science room can be viewed by the pupils of other classes and comparisons made. The ability to evaluate has to be taught, as the pupils find it difficult to compare, contrast and judge. Classifying objects, information or results is also a problem. Predicting outcomes and drawing conclusions are abstract skills requiring practice and encouragement. Variations in results can be difficult for dyslexic children to identify and explain. Skills of generalization and evaluation are not strengths for many of the dyslexic population as observations are taken literally and any finer nuances may be missed. The dyslexic child may not see why further exploration or explanation is necessary.

USE OF TEXT BOOKS

Specific text books are used in the teaching of topics. They are read together as a group activity. The pupils are shown how to find information from the texts, the pictures and diagrams. Dyslexic pupils have more difficulty than is usual in being able to select relevant passages for information and in paraphrasing, as they cannot determine which words or phrases are the most important. Because they have reading problems they often struggle to decode the words and cannot simultaneously practise more advanced literacy skills. Following a sequence of instructions creates possibilities for confusion, with dyslexic pupils muddling up the order or missing out a vital stage altogether.

PRACTICAL ASSIGNMENTS

A 'hand-on' approach to topic assignments has always been a popular and successful method for covering work in conventional schools. For dyslexic pupils it assumes even greater validity. Following multisensory methods of listening, seeing and doing makes the children more motivated because they are actively involved in what they are learning. They benefit in trying things out for themselves, working out methods by trial and error, working in pairs and groups to prove or disprove theories, learning from their mistakes, preparing facts and results for verbal presentation and discussion and developing skills for writing down conclusions.

SCIENCE

In science, pupils are encouraged to plan their experiments, locating the necessary equipment themselves, and to work with care, accuracy and safety. Ingenuity with materials can produce interesting experiments. The pupils are taught how to record their science work using headings which give the pupils a structure to work to. They write the title, followed by the equipment required, the method and the results, finishing with the conclusion and a diagram. When the children have learned to use a word processor, a standard format for recording experiments can be stored in the individual pupil's disc. Account will need to be taken of the problems of the dyspraxic child, who may need to be given more space to work and whose clumsiness must be tolerated.

HOLIDAY PROJECTS

Pupils continue their topic work, extend their general knowledge and develop new areas of interest during the holidays by producing 'projects'. These involve research, planning, organization, writing and presentational skills. The pupils are able to gain practice in these skills and consolidate their knowledge. Results are often very rewarding. These projects replace holiday tasks more specifically related to curriculum subjects, which the children often find demotivating and boring.

VISUAL REINFORCEMENT

In history, a sense and concept of time is fostered in the children by the construction of time lines. Time is an abstract concept and sequencing is often a problem. Visual aids help to develop an awareness of this concept. Historical reconstruction, visits to appropriate museums or sites all bring concrete reality to what can be a puzzling area of knowledge for dyslexic pupils.

By constructively sketching a map in a geography lesson while the teacher is reading out the relevant information, a pupil may take in a lot more about the place than by copying a paragraph from a book about it. The pupil is also being kept active in the learning process. Each topic will have a number of key words in geography which are an essential part of that topic. These will be used in the library for finding information in books or from the CD-ROM. Geography is a good means of transmitting and practising study skills which dyslexic pupils need to acquire if they are to survive in a mainstream classroom and access the full curriculum. Map work can help improve directional and orientation skills.

Study skills help the acquisition and retention of useful and valuable knowledge, bring together facts in their proper context and foster the ability to use and construct visual and graphic materials and models, improving written work and vocabulary. Selectivity is important, with the pupils able to understand the relevance of certain materials. As they are relatively slower at many tasks than other children, they must learn to prioritize.

Teaching information technology

Information technology has been shown to be a very successful medium for dyslexic pupils. Word processors offer considerable help, as they allow the children to amend their writing before the final draft is printed. There is an increase in motivation to write for many children, because the final copy is neat and legible (no handwriting errors) and accurate (fewer spelling worries if the spell check is used).

TOUCH TYPING

Touch typing is taught in the senior part of the school as a preliminary skill to using the word processors properly. Touch typing will never develop naturally and if children are to learn competent touch typing there must be considerable investment of time and effort. For dyslexic children a multisensory, sequential, literacy-based approach is needed, whereby each letter position is learned and practised using common letter strings. It should be tightly structured and proceed from single letters to letter strings to words and then to phrases. Such skills are best taught over a defined and limited period of at least a term, with half-hour lessons on a daily basis. Fairley House has produced its own touch-typing programme based on cumulative phonic principles and with extensive visual and auditory reinforcements. Children keep an ongoing record of their progress and is ensured success through the intentionally gradual introduction of new patterns, which is very motivating.

Many dyslexic children have difficulty identifying patterns. By typing out letter strings they are using another sense, touch. They can feel their fingers following a similar pattern in each group of words and they will build up a vocabulary of these word patterns. A clear example of this is 'was', which forms a triangle on the left hand side of the keyboard. Some children remember these patterns because, after completing the course, children have been seen tapping out words in the air when they are writing in their books and are not sure of a spelling.

To foster kinaesthetic feedback, the children's fingers and keyboards are covered with a cardboard box, which obscures the keyboard but leaves the hands free. A plan of the keyboard on each screen shows the keys learned and this helps the children to find them by touch. Having to find the keys without seeing them and relying to a great extent on kinaesthetic feedback provides the children with a more secure knowledge of the keyboard.

Initially the children are encouraged to say the letters out loud as they type. This auditory reinforcement strengthens the multisensory elements of the operation. Visual reinforcement is supplied through colour coding on the screen, so that all the letters covered by any one finger have the same colour. This colour is used only on the letters that have already been learned, avoiding confusion.

It is more beneficial to focus on accuracy first and allow for speed to develop with knowledge. Children need to be encouraged to develop precision and care. Positive reinforcement techniques are incorporated throughout lessons.

A pilot study

During the pilot study, pupils were tested after several weeks. One 9-year-old child was able to touch-type at 15 w.p.m. and even the weakest child increased his speed significantly. The foundations had been very soundly laid on which the children could build up their speed and accuracy.

LAPTOP WORD PROCESSORS

An initial short-term goal for using laptops was to motivate children and enable those with severe handwriting difficulties to keep pace with their classmates in their production of legible written work. Normally dyslexic children with weak fine motor skills may have to spend a large proportion of study time concentrating on their handwriting in order to make it legible. Using a laptop, they can spend more time on the content. A laptop is ideal for the child whose stronger learning channel is verbal. Children who have problems with far- or near-point copying no longer need to take their eye off the text if they can touch type accurately, so are less likely to lose their place.

The focus is not only on the dyslexic pupil with severe handwriting problems, but on all dyslexic children. Laptop word processors give a boost to the pupil's self-esteem, due to the professional presentation. They give freedom from worry about weak spelling, which can be helped by the spell check facility. They also strengthen the pupils' organizational skills. These are generally improved through the management of the laptops. A pupil's concentration can also improve when using a laptop. Because both hands are busy on the machine, there is no temptation to fiddle.

Use of laptop word processors

Teachers encourage the use of laptops in the classroom in many different ways. Pupils can use laptops for spelling tests and dictation, where their speed increases to keep pace with faster oral input. This is good practice for future notetaking. The laptop opens up a whole new area of study skills.

The portability of the laptop is a great advantage. It is light enough to be carried easily and can be used for homework, helping the pupils to manage their laptops independently, as well as for classwork instead of a pencil and paper. When work has been printed, it is simple for the children to edit, especially if double spacing has been used. It is beneficial to have a printer readily available, as delay causes frustration and limits the practical use of the laptop.

The spell check can release dyslexic children from the fear they often have of writing down an incorrect spelling. The more children produce well-spelled, legible work, the more likely they are to improve their literacy skills. The more the pupils use correctly spelled words, the better their spelling will become. A spell check is ideal for dyslexic pupils if it highlights and bleeps at a wrong spelling. Often when children know which word is wrong, they can correct it for themselves. They are also saved from doubting their own correct spellings. Children with learning disabilities are quite efficient at recognizing the correct spelling from the list offered. Spell checks are suitable for children whose reading is at the 8½-year level or above and is significantly better than their spelling.

Teaching physical education (PE) and games

Gross motor skills are remediated in physical education (PE), games and motor class. Children learn co-ordination. They are made aware of body image, orientation, directionality, spatial awareness and eye–hand coordination. They learn to work together in pairs or as a group. Listening skills are fostered as they must remember instructions and act upon them.

POSSIBLE PROBLEMS

A number of dyslexic pupils have organizational problems and forget to bring their PE clothes into school on the correct day. They may lose them in the school and have no idea how to locate the missing items. While getting changed some dyspraxic pupils have difficulty in undressing or dressing with buttons and shoelaces and with the order in which to put on the clothes. They cannot remember where they put their clothes and will put on the nearest pair of shorts, assuming that they belong to them.

Some pupils cannot follow instructions and are easily confused during an activity. The vocabulary of each game played is different and the children often become confused. Specific terms such as 'bail' or 'wicket' must be explained. Games which have a sequential theme can be a problem, with pupils missing out a stage or muddling them up. Games which involve directional skills can be puzzling to pupils with directional difficulties.

Many of the dyslexic pupils have played games in the past without understanding what the game was about and have been unable to perceive what is going to happen next. A further difficulty with a number of pupils is that when they achieve a certain skill in a game they try to dominate, unaware of the team element. All these difficulties have led to failure in the past and many pupils do not enjoy games until they have a strong sense of both the rules and the ethos of the game. Dyspraxic children who are clumsy and poorly co-ordinated may have always been the last to be picked for teams and be demoralized by games as a result of this.

MOTOR CLASS

Motor class is an activity in small groups for children who need to develop their gross motor skills. Upper limb strengthening exercises involve the building up of shoulder muscles. Many of the games and activities involve the building up of muscle tone, developing the skills needed for balance, such as plenty of movement and change of direction. The children are encouraged to use their own ideas for problem solving and how to overcome their own weaknesses. They find this very rewarding and it helps develop their self-esteem and self-confidence.

Teaching design technology (DT)

Design technology (DT) is an increasingly important lesson for all children, developing skills which are vital in modern life. Using simple design skills, tools and basic materials, children learn how mechanisms work and how they are put together, by making three-dimensional models in a fully equipped workshop. Dyspraxic pupils may find it difficult to plan a task in technology and then execute the project. Children are given the opportunity in these classes to improve their fine motor skills through cutting, drawing, pasting and measurement. They must judge distances, assemble, predict effects and learn through trial and error. Putting the tools and equipment away in its allotted place at the end of a lesson is a useful exercise in organization, memory and co-ordination.

The emphasis in DT is on the practical nature of the task and the lesson centres around problem solving and in thinking in three dimensions. Design technology involves a large degree of craft. The DT projects are planned to relate to the termly topic, so that work in technology can complement science, maths or topic work.

Throughout the academic year, children are given the opportunity to work independently, pacing their own work alongside their peers, discovering their own standard of quality and their own problems confronting tools and materials. Later in the year they will embark on a group project. Many factors of group work have to be dealt with: the delegation of tasks, the assembling of one object from parts made by several different groups, establishment of roles within the group and negotiation about the work the group expects from each individual. This is excellent for developing oral language skills and fosters listening and communication skills.

There are always children who cannot cope with a lively, unstructured class, with the noise and energy of hammering, drilling and discussion that characterizes a DT workshop. If they are naturally distractible, they become more so, finding these conditions only aggravate their problems. They react by exploiting the informality of the workshop, by being disruptive, complaining of nausea or headaches. Others do not like to touch and use certain textures like clay and need help to overcome these feelings by Occupational Therapists using desensitization techniques. These children are discreetly 'specialled' by staff, given extra time, help and support.

Most children will learn the basics of woodwork, measuring and cutting timber, using a bench drill and a glue gun. They will assemble accurate models cut from card or plastic using Stanley knives, scissors and metal rulers. They will work with electric cable, batteries, bulbs and switches, gears and electric motors. They will make models from recycled materials. The children evaluate the success of their projects by making graphs, filling in questionnaires and comparing their projects with those of other groups, classes or individuals. The topic-related language skills acquired will be of importance in later life.

It is important to consider the range of abilities in a DT lesson and children can learn a great deal from each other. They will be rewarded for a helpful, cooperative attitude, specially for sharing skills with those less able, while they may achieve a boost in confidence from the help they offered.

Dyslexic children are often original and imaginative. They find, however, that their imagination runs ahead of their capability to implement their ideas. They can become very frustrated with their own personal limits and can be impatient when they discover they have to do things more than once. Children, on the whole, find DT very satisfying and they are proud to have an end product to show to parents, teachers, siblings and friends. The ideal DT project will foster independent learning skills.

Teaching art

It is perhaps instinctive to assume that art is an area where dyslexic children would have no problems. Dyslexic children can seem more successful at art and a teacher may inadvertently demand less accuracy from a drawing than from a written account. Slowness and care taken over the lines of a drawing are seen as strengths in an art lesson while a similar approach to notetaking is regarded in a different light. Standards are less rigid and the criteria by which the finished product is judged less obvious.

Art is seen as a release from the pressures of a normal school day. It is relatively unstructured and in a different room. The register of the language used in art is quite different from other lessons. The children usually chat about subjects of their own choosing and with little censure. Art is rarely a collective strength. Some pupils will always show initial and sometimes extreme resistance to drawing and painting, assuming that whatever they draw will be bad. Pictures communicate very directly. A child can see errors or failings in their pictures far more quickly than they may register errors in written work.

The fine motor control needed in an art lesson can also be a problem. Responding to different mediums takes fine adjustments in the handling of paint brushes, chalks, pastels or pencils. Drawing hinges on the quality and range of line produced by these materials.

Children tend to draw what they predict they will see, rather than what they actually see. Drawing a still life demands a great deal of the pupil's power of memory. The repeated movements of the eye from the observed object to the drawing paper can be laborious and non-instinctive. For a dyslexic child with a short concentration span and low self-esteem, the motivation to experiment and persevere may be lacking and little of any value will be produced.

Drawings of complex, imagined or remembered objects rely on the student's experience of and interest in them. A child may draw in order of importance or recall and often from memories which are only partial. These pupils have an episodic grasp of reality; they see bits but not the whole. They do not register the importance of the main structures of an object.

PLANNING AND ORGANIZATION

Planning can be important to help children who feel discouraged about the images they produce. Talking through a picture before and after it is drawn can be helpful. Group and self-assessment of lessons can provide an opportunity for children to express their feelings about a task, discussing what was fun and what was difficult; it also allows them to accept praise, encouragement and criticism from their peers.

From an organizational point of view, it is often difficult for children to predict and remember what materials they may need for a task. The cleaning and storing of those materials after use is again challenging. Art provides an opportunity to tackle a pupil's personal organization. Lessons run far more smoothly, however, if the basics of paper, medium and brush can be set up before the lesson begins. The pupils are then responsible for choosing, finding and tidying away any additional materials they might need.

Art lessons provide an opportunity to involve all the senses in work and can be used to reinforce ideas and issues covered in other subjects. Art provides excellent opportunities for remediation.

Teaching drama

Drama gives the children the chance to express their feelings without hindrance, allowing them to release their frustrations by voicing their emotions in a safe and controlled environment. Many pupils have a natural talent in this area which surprises teachers, parents and even the children themselves. Any confidence gained in drama has a knock-on effect in other areas of their education, encouraging them to experiment, creating a positive learning cycle. Naturally shy children can hide behind a character and use drama as a vessel to convey their ideas and feelings.

Communication skills are developed and relate to the speech and language of the dyslexic child. The use of verbal exercises and games helps to build vocabulary, strengthen the children's understanding of sentence structure and develop conversational skills. Drama ties in closely with the work of the Occupational Therapists, incorporating balance, coordination and spatial awareness to enhance muscle control and body discipline.

Drama also provides an opportunity to build friendships and the sense of belonging to a group, by emphasizing the importance of each individual member's contribution in producing a successful piece of group work. It promotes self-image and confidence, public speaking, voice projection, audience awareness, team and partner work and body orientation. An annual play can provide an excellent opportunity for cooperative achievement. A number of dyslexic children exhibit a high standard of acting. Learning roles can be difficult for some pupils, but these children can have their lines put on tape so that they can listen to them daily. High levels of motivation are also an important factor for learning lines.

The classes can produce whole group stories and drama improvizations through partner work. This is achieved through setting a problem which, through imaginative analysis and discussion, the group can solve and act out.

Perhaps the most important aspect of drama lessons is the contribution made to the children's ability to express themselves clearly and being able to give an oral presentation in order to communicate. This can be especially important for interviews.

Teaching music

Conventional approaches to teaching the subject need to be adapted for dyslexic pupils with the emphasis lying in the strategies used to increase the pupils' skills of organization, sociability and listening.

The importance of rhythm, sequencing and turn taking cannot be stressed enough. Many dyslexic children experience difficulties with various aspects of music, including the language. For instance concepts of 'higher' and 'lower' may be poorly understood. Musical notation is another form of symbolic representation which may cause problems. Rhythm work is particularly useful to help pupils with poor motor coordination and weak planning skills. This area is reinforced when the children play instruments, learn to conduct or compose their own music.

Many children with poor spatial skills have difficulty discriminating pitch and singing in tune. Games and exercises are devised to develop this skill. A multisensory approach can be used and most lessons incorporate movement into the music. Children learn to read basic music, beginning with composing simple music themselves. A sense of rhythm, which can be taught through music, is very helpful for dyslexic children. Some dyslexic children have weaknesses with hand–eye coordination and some experience confusion over direction. A lot of work involves clapping, stamping, slapping and tapping out rhythms. Also, since they may have considerable difficulty keeping their own tune or rhythm against another, a lot of rounds are sung.

It is beneficial to emphasize singing, humming and pitch discrimination. The latter in particular can cause real difficulties. Dyslexics often take longer to establish an inner sense of pitch. They often have a poor awareness of external space and therefore show directional confusion, while those who have a strong sense of space tend to be able to sing in tune. Few know even the most common nursery rhymes and rhyming songs. Since rhythm relates to spelling, the ability to recognize sound patterns in words can be extremely useful. Another interesting feature is that, as confidence increases, so their sense of pitch improves. Other areas of emphasis are the use of dynamics both with vocal and instrumental work (they sometimes have difficulty judging volume), conducting (excellent for laterality and directionality confusion) and listening skills, where they can be trained to listen for particular sounds. Musical terminology can be discussed and confusions are put right.

The pattern of difficulties is varied but clear-cut. The children's achievements as musicians are affected by the problems of having to read notation as more time is needed for symbolic processing. Awareness of theory may suffer through weak memory skills, a lack of understanding of the underlying concept or simply through poor handwriting skills. Concepts such as high and low and loud and soft are sometimes difficult and there can be confusion over labelling; many musical terms are in Italian. Weaknesses in the fine motor skills may hamper the 'delivery' of a piece of music. Dyslexics have difficulty establishing a sense of rhythm.

They may also experience difficulty over left and right, confusing which hand to use when playing an instrument.

A thorough auditory and visual training is helpful in providing a basis upon which to learn an instrument. Practical musical skills, learning to process sounds or to follow a pattern of symbols can be given a special focus in initial lessons.

An awareness of sound is fundamental and work is done in discriminating sounds, listening for patterns in the music and engaging in various kinds of aural exercises. Training in rhythm skills helps poor coordination. Rhythm work can also be integrated into motor classes taken by the Occupational Therapists.

Theory is potentially a problem area and must be explained by means of the sounds which the symbols or words represent. If the theory is integrated with auditory skills early on, then its relevance is clear. It is important that theory serves as a means to record and communicate different sounds and that its importance is not overestimated.

Music can be of value as a remedial tool as learning takes place in a 'fun' activity, involving something new in terms of symbol discrimination. The child is not being 'remediated' by means of a language which embodies struggle, frustration and memories of failure. It stimulates the imagination and as an expressive outlet it has great value. There are also some dyslexic pupils who are gifted musically and have exceptional abilities. Their talent not only enhances their self-esteem but is a great emotional release.

Homework policy

Homework is given to all children regardless of their age. The very young children begin by getting into the routine of reading aloud to an adult each evening. By the age of seven most children have to read and learn their lists of words for spelling. Older pupils may also have to complete some kind of written work. This may be finishing off work begun in class or may be a reinforcement activity following on from something covered in class that day or week. The main emphasis is to encourage the children to settle down independently at home, with responsibility for their own work. Parents are encouraged to settle their child in a regular, quiet place with any resources the child may require readily available, but then to withdraw to allow the child to work alone for a set amount of time. Both parent and child know that the child is answerable to the teacher for the work produced, thus avoiding stress and tension within the family. Homework diaries can be used to ensure contact between the parent and the class teacher and as a reminder to the pupils of the content of each evening's task.

Even though the homework routine is structured and appropriate, it can easily break down. Dyslexic children are often more tired at the end of the school day. Parents may not be at home to ensure that homework is completed and these children are no exception in wriggling out of commitments if any excuse can be found. It is, however, essential that homework is conscientiously completed and that the plea 'I can't do it because I am dyslexic' does not win exemption.

Teaching modern foreign languages

When pupils reach secondary school they are expected to learn at least one foreign language. Many dyslexics have trouble coping with the reading, spelling, grammar and specialist vocabulary of their own language. So much time and effort is put into learning English, where progress can be slow and skills achieved with difficulty, that it could be unfair to burden the dyslexic pupil with another language. If learning is confined to conversation, then some may make progress without too much difficulty, but one must be aware that the dyslexic pupil may become more confused and frustrated than their non-dyslexic peer. Italian and Spanish would possibly be easier to learn than French.

Summary

Dyslexic children whose problems are severe enough to need a period of total immersion will require a different teaching style and class teachers who have a clear understanding of their pupils' difficulties throughout the school day. Class teachers must apply remedial techniques to every aspect of the curriculum to ensure that these children do not miss out on their broader education.

For maximum success, therefore, it is essential that all the teachers involved with these pupils should have obtained specialist remedial qualifications in the teaching of children with specific learning difficulties. Ongoing training is also important. Close contact with the Educational Psychologist, the Speech and Language Therapists, the Occupational Therapists and the remedial teachers, as with the other professionals involved with the welfare of the child, ensures a holistic approach to the dyslexic child's problems. It provides better opportunities for ensuring that remedial intervention will be successful and that transfer back into mainstream education will be a realistic target. The teaching of dyslexic children is a stimulating challenge and can be most rewarding and exciting for both pupils and teachers.

References

Cox, A.R. (1977) *Situation Spelling*, Educators Publishing Service, Cambridge, Mass.
Fernald, G.M. (1943) *Remedial Techniques on Basic School Subjects*, McGraw-Hill, New York.

Further reading

Miles, T.R. and Miles, E. (eds) (1992) *Dyslexia and Mathematics*, Routledge, London.
Pollock, J. and Waller, E. (1994) *Day-to-day Dyslexia in the Classroom*, Routledge, London.

10 *The Headteacher*

Patience Thomson

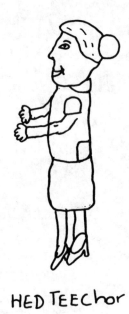

HED TEEChor

Fig. 10.1 The Headteacher as seen by a dyslexic child.

A whole school approach

THE OVERVIEW

The Headteacher must coordinate the functions of all those associated with the school. This will at times include working with those outside the teaching or medical profession – the school governors, architects, builders, lawyers, the social services or occasionally the media. It involves working with the professional experts brought in for consultation, such as the Orthoptist, Paediatrician and School Counsellor. The main emphasis of the Headteacher's role will, however, focus on close involvement with staff, parents and children.

The remedial support afforded the dyslexic pupil in a mainstream school is often fragmented. Those who provide it will only see part of the picture. The Educational Psychologist, Speech and Language Therapist, Occupational Therapist, specialist remedial teacher or School Counsellor may see the child on or off site. In either situation it is unlikely that any of them will have a holistic view of how the child is functioning on a day-to-day basis in the classroom, in the unstructured situations of the school day or at home. Although the remedial teacher is more likely to operate on site, with better contact, such help is often provided on a peripatetic basis, with little time scheduled for communication with the other professionals. Written reports are no substitute for daily personal contact and regular discussion.

Yet it is vitally important that the professionals should confer for two reasons. First, it will have become apparent from the previous chapters that the complexity and diversity of specific learning difficulties require expert diagnosis and management, involving a wide range of expertise. Second, and just as important, is the need to act quickly to resolve the problems of dyslexic children before the gap which separates them from their classmates widens into a daunting chasm. The sense of urgency must be maintained if the child is to acquire as quickly as possible the level of competence in basic literacy and numeracy skills required to function normally in a conventional mainstream classroom. The necessary progress can only be achieved by designing for each child an individual education plan which will draw in the professional experts, as and when they are needed, at each stage of the process. If all these professionals are available on site this is much easier to coordinate. In the case of the visiting consultants, the Paediatrician, the Orthoptist and the School Counsellor, opportunities must be sought for them to speak directly to staff whenever necessary. The Headteacher must act as an intermediary and coordinator to ensure that they are fully briefed on each child.

The Headteacher must also dedicate a considerable amount of time to the initial assessment of children to ensure that the right pupils are admitted to the school. A wrong choice is not only disadvantageous to the child but also puts unwarranted pressure on all the professionals involved. This is particularly true of aggressive children or of those with pronounced behavioural problems. Although all the professionals involved in the assessment procedures will advise as to suitability, the Headteacher must make the final decision in each individual case.

THE ETHOS OF THE SCHOOL

What the Headteacher must determine, establish and maintain is the ethos of the school. In a school for dyslexic children this will include decisions on priorities, in terms of the curriculum and timetable, resources and staff. It will also entail the setting of realistic goals for the school, staff, parents and individual children. This cannot be done in isolation. The participation of all the experts involved with the school is needed. Attitudes must be positive and dyslexia must be viewed by the staff as a challenge and not a handicap if the long hours, the temporary frustrations and setbacks and the constant effort required to produce an intensive and supportive programme are not to affect their commitment and morale. Longer term strategy planning must not be crowded out by the incessant demands of the weekly timetable.

A sense of purpose can be gained from the belief that dyslexics can be high achievers if enabled to develop their own individual talents. Of late, much attention has been drawn to the achievements of dyslexics in many fields. This has been particularly well documented by West (1991) who has examined the effects of learning difficulties on the creative lives of such diverse subjects as Albert Einstein, Lewis Carroll, Michael Faraday and Winston Churchill. Moreover, Gardner (1983) has questioned previous definitions of intelligence as identified in standardized tests and has developed the concept of multiple intelligences. These, according to his view, include linguistic intelligence, musical intelligence, logical-mathematical intelligence, spatial intelligence, bodily-kinaesthetic intelligence and personal intelligences.

Personal intelligences include interpersonal skills, or the ability to relate to other people and to understand relationships, and intrapersonal skills, or self-analysis, which is the ability to understand one's own character, behaviour, feelings and thought processes. Since skills and therefore talent in any of these areas can bring dividends in terms of self-respect and success in life, education in its broadest sense should foster in each child their strengths wherever they may lie.

Children will have divergent potential in these different areas and no individual will be uniformly endowed in all the six identified 'intelligences'. It therefore follows that no one method of teaching will be appropriate to every pupil. For this reason it is an important basic premise that the child who fails to understand what has to be learned is not 'stupid', but may require the information to be presented differently. The teacher must lift the burden of guilt or distress from the child who feels frustrated because he or she cannot learn and adapt the teaching style until the child can and does learn. This flexibility of approach is fundamental to an effective school policy.

In discussion with parents, staff or children I often talk about the 'aha' and the 'wow' factors and to my mind these are essential ingredients of a successful approach to lifting the barriers to learning and development which dyslexia inevitably creates. The 'aha' factor relates to the understanding and insight which staff, parents and children should gain as individual problems are identified and strategies or solutions put into effect. The 'wow' factor is the astonishment on all fronts when these children achieve at a level which is not just 'very good for a dyslexic' or an improvement on past performance, but excellent by any standards. Sam was a case in point.

Sam (15)

Sam was school phobic. He came to me for a remedial session once a week at the Dyslexia Clinic at St Bartholomew's Hospital. He had been assessed by the Clinical Psychologist there as being of above average intelligence. The aim was to ease him back gradually into mainstream school, starting with a few lessons a week. I ascertained that the only subject which had fired his imagination at school was biology, possibly because he had a teacher who was young, pretty and sympathetic. We set, as our target, that he should sit GCSE biology. To this end his mother, Sam and I compiled a set of index cards covering the syllabus. We used colour coding, diagrams and mind maps and kept any written notes as brief as possible. We numbered the index cards and divided them into manageable sections. We checked with his teacher in case of doubt. Sam was involved at every stage, prompting, participating and incidentally learning the facts as the project grew. The result was a work of art and we were all proud of it.

Then came the school holidays and a temporary suspension of the sessions. It was two months before I saw Sam again. He produced his cards and my heart sank. They were dog-eared and torn. Some were missing. Others were scribbled over, some with graffiti-type messages. My distress turned to anger and, forgetting my role as a sympathetic and understanding remedial therapist, I berated Sam soundly. He listened quietly and then he grinned, 'Mrs T., I've been hiring out these cards for a couple of quid a time and I've made a fortune'.

The 'aha' factor was that in the course of the exercise not only Sam, but his mother, his teacher and I learned a great deal about study skills and how to apply them. Our strategies worked and light dawned for Sam. The 'wow' factor was not just that, through our mutual efforts, we achieved a creditable result, but that Sam's peers were suitably impressed by what he had done and his self-esteem restored.

Praise from parents or teachers can appear suspect. Children are all too aware that encouragement from these sources may be related to a perceived need for praise and not to actual levels of performance. Admiration and acknowledgement from contemporaries, on the other hand, have real value to a child. The 'aha' factor affords insight and the 'wow' factor increases self-confidence. Both are essential ingredients if dyslexic children are to maintain their motivation and set themselves high standards.

What is true for the individual is true for a school. If staff are trying out new approaches, learning new skills, adapting their teaching style and analysing problems with a view to finding solutions, there is a constant 'aha' factor as they realize which strategies are proving successful. The 'wow' factor must come from the world outside when the products of the system are evaluated objectively and approved.

RECORD KEEPING

There is undeniably more paperwork to be dealt with in a specialist school. Precise and detailed records need to be kept for every child. Every meeting and every telephone call must be documented. At the time of the child's initial assessment there will often be a considerable volume of reports to consider. An important source of information is the detailed questionnaire containing background information about the medical and educational history of the child, including the parents' perception of the problems involved. It must be carefully scrutinized, as must any records from previous schools and relevant professional reports. The regular individual reviews and reports which are sent out to parents and local education authorities (LEAs) must be more frequent and more detailed than would be necessary for children without learning difficulties. A close check must be kept on the progress of every child.

INFORMATION GATHERING

Time must be found to read the current literature and keep in touch with new developments in the field. Much research to determine the nature and establish the causes of the various manifestations of dyslexia is currently being undertaken, both in Britain and abroad. Representatives of many professional disciplines are involved. Attending conferences and seminars, where theoretical issues are discussed, provides the Headteacher and other senior members of staff with information which may well affect practical policy. All the staff benefit from the cross-fertilization of ideas afforded by the visits of outside professionals to the school and through time spent visiting other establishments. Insularity or self-satisfaction is particularly dangerous in a climate where perceptions are shifting all the time.

ALLOCATION OF RESOURCES

Close consultation with the staff is essential if necessary resource material is to be acquired. It is the Headteacher's task to enable the members of the multidisciplinary team to function effectively within the school setting and to see that they have the proper working environment and adequate resources. It is also important to prevent any duplication in the provision offered and to see that no obvious area of weakness has been overlooked. Priorities must be established.

Typical examples can be cited. It was the urgent request of the Occupational Therapist that the children should all have desks which were easily adjustable as to height and writing slope. This constituted a major capital outlay. Two classes were given them as a pilot scheme to establish what benefit they afforded. It emerged that vulnerable children with poor muscular control were enabled to maintain a far better body posture while working, could concentrate for longer and found the physical effort of writing less stressful. Such was the success of these desks that their use was extended to the whole school.

Computers are unfortunately very expensive, but they are a high priority because they are instrumental in improving motivation, self-confidence and performance. When purchasing computers for educational purposes, it should be borne in mind that the expense is not confined to the initial purchase of hardware. Requirements grow for improved software, new programs and CD-ROMs and, as general competence improves, there are demands for more sophisticated and updated equipment. An often forgotten factor is the ongoing need for all the staff to be trained to make full use of the facilities offered. If staff feel threatened and fearful that their lack of knowledge will be revealed, they will not encourage the children to make full use of their laptops or the facilities of the computer room and expensive equipment will lie idle. Forward planning is necessary to ensure that continuing funds are made available.

Another outlay which was given top priority by the staff, with the backing of the governing body, was the acquisition of enough laptop word processors to equip the top five classes in the school. Again a pilot scheme confirmed that the models chosen were appropriate to children of this age, that they were sturdy enough for everyday use and that they could and would be used on a daily basis. It was essential to monitor that this actually happened in practice.

Not having to share books or equipment is an important factor if maximum intensive benefit is to be derived from lessons. Since the curriculum must be modified and since differentiated materials are required for children with learning difficulties, this is bound to involve considerable expense. Some items, such as carpets in the classroom which might be regarded as a luxury, are surprisingly important for dyslexic children. They significantly improve the working environment by reducing noise levels and hence distractions for the child who has problems with maintaining concentration and attention levels.

STAFF CONTACT

It is under the direction of the Headteacher that the roles and responsibilities of the various members of staff are established. Regular contact with the staff through formal and informal meetings each week is important. Whenever possible, the 'open door' policy means that staff have ready access. Informal visits to the classroom and to remedial sessions enable the Headteacher to have a general overall view of how both the curriculum and the remedial programme are being delivered.

STAFF TRAINING

Staff training is an essential ingredient if everyone on site is to work for the maximum benefit of the child. The remedial help offered is highly specialized and the approach adopted by the various disciplines, Speech and Language Therapists, Occupational Therapists, remedial teachers and classteachers can be very different. In-service workshops should be arranged so that the professionals can demonstrate their work to each other. Training is also needed for others on site who may have considerable contact with the children but who have no formal training, such as the team of class assistants and the office staff. If they have some knowledge of the rationale behind the teaching and remedial approaches, their jobs become more interesting and effective. It is important, for instance, that class assistants should know that a child with poor receptive language skills may not respond immediately to instructions. Again, the school secretaries may need to know that a child with weak expressive language skills may be unable to explain why they are feeling unwell. They often need infinite patience in the office to unravel a message from a parent relayed through a child. It is the job of the Headteacher not only to see that staff training is timetabled, but also to ensure that it is not abandoned because of the day-to-day pressures of school life.

Working with parents

COMMUNICATION

The Headteacher must be readily available for parents, as they are very much part of the team. There is much they can do to reinforce and support the school programme, but they will need explanation and encouragement. Problems on the home front can easily affect school performance and any information of this nature needs to be passed on to all those involved with the child. As Vivienne McKennell, the School Counsellor, has described in her chapter, the death of a beloved pet, even short absences of one or both parents, the departure of a carer, the birth of a new baby or any alteration to a mother's or father's work routine can temporarily disconcert any child. Dyslexics, who seem to adapt less easily to change, may often display exaggerated negative reactions.

Michael (9)
Michael's work went sharply downhill almost overnight, his concentration deteriorated and he became moody, lethargic and silent. Much effort was expended in exploring possible causes within the school framework. It was then discovered by chance that the interior of his house was being repainted and he had been turned out of his bedroom. He hated the disruption, the smell and the chaos. After six weeks, order was restored at home and progress picked up at school.

Prompt communication, a note or telephone call from the parents to the school, saves much time otherwise spent fruitlessly searching for underlying reasons for a child's distress or lack of performance.

If parents are to be effectively involved in supporting the child's remedial programme, it is important to give them confidence by explaining exactly what is required. It has been mentioned that dyslexia is often inherited, so one or other of the parents may have dyslexic problems themselves. It is particularly important, therefore, that any written communications with parents should be clear and jargon-free and that they should be followed up with oral explanations if required. Everyone involved, teachers, therapists and office staff, needs to listen carefully, to repeat themselves where necessary and to respect and understand the anxieties and concerns of the parents, many of whom will be tense when discussing their child.

A useful guide to parents who wish to find out more about dyslexia is *Overcoming Dyslexia* (Hornsby, 1984). Hornsby points out that 'It is not possible to give parents definitive, step-by-step guidelines that are guaranteed to lead to success, as each child will respond differently to whatever is done to help' and goes on to say, 'Be prepared for your child to be unresponsive to the help you offer'. These are practical words of wisdom. Ostler (1991) has also written a book full of constructive advice for parents.

Emotion clouds the ability to make sense of information and can lead to misinterpretations. These should be expected and preempted wherever possible. Parents of dyslexic children can become distressed in their search for solutions. Feelings of inadequacy and guilt are not uncommon, particularly as the causes of dyslexia are not clearly understood. The fact that it is often hereditary may lead one or other parent to regard it as their 'fault'. Other causes are less obvious and parents question their management skills. They reproach themselves that the problems were not recognized earlier and appropriate help provided. They suspect that they have been unsympathetic, overprotective, underprotective or generally inadequate.

There are facets of dyslexia which parents find baffling and frustrating, such as their child's inability to remember next day the spelling list or tables which were learned so painfully for homework the evening before. Dyslexics lose things, break things, forget things and confuse things. Other manifestations   such as clumsiness, disorganization, particularly where personal effects are concerned, failure to remember instructions or the inability to maintain friendships may not necessarily have been associated with a specific learning difficulty until the child is diagnosed as dyslexic or dyspraxic.

When the parents learn, at the initial assessment from the multi-disciplinary team, the true nature and extent of their child's difficulties, there is often a sense of relief. They then need explanation of what the diagnosis implies and of how the problems will be addressed. They need to be instructed with clear guidelines as to their part in supporting the remedial programme. They can then return to their true role of parenting, which should include prime enjoyment and recreation time with their children. Too often the hours spent with their dyslexic child had previously been dedicated to accompanying them to regular sessions with different specialists, helping with homework or chivvying them to accomplish the very tasks which caused most difficulty.   No wonder parent–child relationships often suffered before help was forthcoming.

SCHOOL REPORTS

If parents are to be realistically informed, school reports must be clear about the criteria by which the child's work has been judged. The child who is top of a maths group in a specialist school setting may well produce a mediocre performance in a mainstream classroom. The true implications of 'remarkable progress' are only meaningful if this is viewed in terms of a clearly established starting point. Again, it is no kindness to parents to omit to mention any problems with behaviour or attitude because there is prevailing sympathy for the child's learning difficulties. As long as suggestions for improvement are included and the positive elements of a child's performance stressed, and as long as all comments are fair and accurate, the 'warts and all' approach can be reassuring and establish trust and confidence between parents and the school.

PARENT–TEACHER MEETINGS

It is helpful if once a year parents can be invited to a meeting with the class teacher at which the child will be present. Samples of work can be shown. If the child has previously conferred with the teacher, they can jointly decide on the areas of strength and weakness to be discussed. Realistic and immediate goals can be set at this meeting. This process proves useful in giving the parent a clear idea of the child's current level of achievement. These meetings, where control lies with the child, can also be a learning experience for all concerned.

HOME MANAGEMENT AND HOMEWORK

Parents should be expected to ensure that children come fresh to school. Late nights watching television, irregular mealtimes or routines, chaotic departure in the morning (particularly if there has been no breakfast), junk food, confrontation and reproach on the doorstep, exhausting weekends away, all impinge seriously on a child's ability to settle down in school and learn effectively. It is advisable for all children to have a regular regime. They should know when they are expected to do homework and have clear space and privacy to get it done. For dyslexic children, who are almost by definition distractible and disorganized, consistent and sensible home management is essential.

Homework is one of the most fraught areas and regular confrontation every evening between children and parents is exhausting and counterproductive. Dyslexic children have a particularly tiring day, even in a school where the curriculum is modified to accommodate their specific needs. This is because they find it difficult to concentrate, are often socially vulnerable and the basic skills which they are learning can only be mastered with considerable effort. Where staff:pupil ratios are high in a specialist school, pupils cannot cruise through the day or daydream at the back of the class. By the time they go home there will be little energy left for academic work. Moreover, bad work habits with regard to homework have probably built up in the past, when they either struggled for hours with little success or were exonerated by a sympathetic teacher who knew that they could not achieve at the same level as their peers.

Holiday homework can be another potential area for acrimonious conflict between parents and children. If the tasks are not properly understood, there is little chance of referring back to teachers, who will be on vacation, and frustration ensues. If the tasks are boring, with repetitive worksheets to fill in, the whole exercise becomes a chore to be completed with the minimum expenditure of time and effort. Regular routines are hard to establish and pervasive guilt can spoil what should be a time for recuperation and relaxation. All too often there is a last-minute scramble before term starts. On the first day of term, the child shamefacedly produces some rushed, ill-digested and poorly presented work. This is counterproductive.

The answer can be the imaginative holiday project. Not only can the choice of topic be relatively free, but the means of presentation can be flexible. Tape recordings, models, collages, shell or pressed flower collections, photographs, pictorial records or computer programs would all be acceptable. Children are expected to supply a title, list of contents, headings and numbered pages. Good organizational skills are extremely important educationally and this is a specific area of weakness for the dyslexic child. Projects provide useful experience.

The projects should be judged on certain clearly stated criteria which must be explained to the pupils and their parents. It is encouraging for children if they have a wide readership. Nothing is more disheartening than spending hours on producing work of a high standard which will only be seen by a classteacher, who will mark it and send it home again. Appropriate arrangements can be made for projects to be seen by all the teachers involved with that child and by classmates. They can also be on view in the school library. Results often provoke the 'wow!' factor, with ingenious and original ways of presenting information. The children inspire each other and are encouraged to improve on their own record with each new project. Parents are initially encouraged to help the child with the planning and execution of these projects, with the choice of subject, with the assembling of material and with the style of presentation. Such support can gradually be withdrawn, but good foundations will hopefully have been laid. Fathers can often be persuaded to be involved, especially if material is gathered on holiday. Mutual enthusiasm for football, windsurfing or geology, for example, can be very therapeutic and a bonding experience. It can also result in a fascinating project.

ORGANIZATION

Many dyslexic children, and most dyspraxic ones, are typically disorganized. A small minority are exceptionally well organized, as if to be obsessively neat was the dike which kept out the sea of chaos threatening to break through at any moment. If children are to be taught organizational skills, this must be done tactfully. Arguments over untidy cupboards, school bags or rooms are not conducive to persuading the child to cooperate. It can be far more positive and enjoyable for the child to start by arranging someone else's possessions, father's or mother's desktop (under supervision!) or the kitchen drawers or cupboards. In categorizing the various types of objects and storing them according to a coherent plan, children learn the underlying rationale of creating a retrieval system. It is likely that these skills, once learned, can be transferred to other areas of the child's life.

LISTENING SKILLS

If children are to acquire effective listening skills, parents must set them a good example. 'Do you think the King knows all about me?' asks Christopher Robin in *When We Were Very Young* (Milne, 1924). 'Sure to, dear, but it's time for tea,' replies Alice, his nanny, quite irrelevantly. How can a child develop communication skills in the face of the 'yes dear, no dear, what did you say dear?' type of response? Great benefits result when one or other parent sets aside time to be alone with the child and to listen quietly, so that the child does not have to compete as they talk against siblings, other adults, the television or the radio.

READING ALOUD

Reading to their children is one of the greatest advantages which parents can offer. For dyslexic children it provides access to a wide range of more challenging literature which they would be unable to read for themselves, although they are mature enough to understand or enjoy the stories and absorb the information. Reading aloud to them familiarizes dyslexic children with the structure and vocabulary of formal written language, which is not the same as spoken language. They will need such understanding if they are to predict or intelligently guess words in context. Finally it introduces children to the authors popular with their peers and siblings, so that they can participate in discussions in class and with family and friends.

Busy parents can record their readings onto a tape. The child can then listen repeatedly and at leisure. Dyslexic children often enjoy such repetition, as their poor listening skills and weak auditory memory may miss much at a first reading. Listening to a tape read by a parent is often a more meaningful experience for the child than listening to the audio tapes available commercially.

CHOOSING THE NEXT SCHOOL – THE VULNERABLE CHILD

Even on the first exploratory visit to the school, parents are often keen to discuss where the children might go on to after a possible two or three year period in an environment which offers intensive help. It should be remembered that while children are moving through the educational process they attend a series of establishments. Staff assume current responsibility for academic input and progress for only a limited period. In the long run, it is the parents who coordinate the various aspects of their children's lives and plan their futures. It is therefore important to help parents acquire practical insight, realistic expectations and an appreciation of current options, if they are to make an informed choice with regard to a child's next school.

However successful the intensive remedial programme appears to be within the sheltered environment of a specialist school, true proof of its effectiveness will only be apparent when the child succeeds, or fails to succeed, to adapt back into mainstream education. In the case of Fairley House, in only a very small minority of cases will a pupil move on to a secondary school which continues to provide intensive remedial help in small groups with such a high staff:pupil ratio. Specialist schools undoubtedly provide a protective environment so parents must be prepared for possible short-term setbacks when their child faces the realities of larger classes and less attention in a mainstream setting. Giving parents and pupils the opportunity to maintain contact with the specialist school they are leaving, especially in the initial period after transfer to a new school, can be most reassuring.

Counselling the parents about future educational provision is essential and this is an area where the Headteacher needs to work closely with the Educational Psychologist. They will together spend much time with parents, having consulted with relevant members of staff, in determining each pupil's current level of functioning. Future needs for remedial support, the type of provision best suited to individual personalities and academic prospects must also be discussed. Where a child has been given a Statement of Special Educational Needs, representatives from the local education authority will normally be present at discussions.

Even with help and guidance, anxiety about the dyslexic child's ability to cope in secondary mainstream education, and the difficulties involved in finding a suitable school which will accept the child, remain a major source of stress for parents.

LOCAL EDUCATION AUTHORITIES (LEAs)

The local education authorities send a small number of children with specific learning difficulties to an independent specialist school for intensive remedial help if there is no suitable provision within the local mainstream schools. Such children will all have a Statement of Special Educational Needs. The whole 'statementing' process, the Code of Practice established by the 1993 Education Act, which is helpfully documented by Russell (1994) and Orton (1994), procedures for monitoring and review, legal implications and possibilities for appeal are complex areas. Parents will need help and support to understand the requirements and to respond appropriately. Appropriate books can be recommended to the parents, such as *Children with Special Needs: Caught in the Act* (Chasty and Friel, 1995), which set out the procedures clearly and succinctly.

The school itself cooperates and works with both the parents and the LEAs at all stages. The initial assessments by the multidisciplinary team are often submitted as contributory evidence. Individual education plans (IEPs), drawn up within the school, are crucial to fulfilling the terms of each individual statement, which will specify precisely what provision is required, including input from the Speech and Language and Occupational Therapists where necessary.

REASSURANCE

Parents who approach a specialist school for help often feel threatened by the implications of dyslexia, by the complexities of the education system and by the difficulties, and in some cases the financial cost, involved in finding the necessary provision for their child. They may react emotionally, either withdrawing beyond the reach of effective support and advice or advancing aggressively to criticize or complain. At every level they need reassurance that their child's problem is being appropriately addressed, that they are being kept fully informed and that, above all, they are not being blamed for their child's difficulties.

Working with children

DIRECT CONTACT

Regular teaching commitments in the classroom, though time consuming for a Headteacher, are important. Without firsthand experience of how the child responds, it is difficult to talk to staff or parents with the depth of insight required to make informed judgements. Contact with the children at their weekly assemblies helps to build up a picture of their personalities and profiles.

A rational and fair disciplinary system within the school is essential, with the ultimate sanction being a visit to the Headteacher. Time must therefore be set aside for seeing children who have misbehaved. Others are sent to the Headteacher for more positive reasons – they have something exciting to show or news to impart. Some individuals may need to be seen because they are upset or worried.

LATERAL THINKERS

Anyone working with dyslexics needs to develop sensitive listening skills. Dyslexic pupils are often unpredictable, lateral thinkers whose conclusions are reached through original channels. It is worthwhile exploring how their minds have been working. Since these children have problems with auditory memory, they are unlikely to repeat verbatim the ideas of others. If they do remember them, it will not be parrot fashion but through processing and understanding the concepts. Information, therefore, often reemerges with a value-added factor of unexpected contribution from the child. Examples of the unusual response are not hard to find.

Gillian (7) and others
Gillian was an exceptionally bright child, yet she could hardly read and her spelling was non-existent. At her assessment, she was asked to relate the story of Noah's Ark. This was to test her ability to sequence ideas coherently. 'God had a problem knowing what to do with the mermaid,' she replied.

The word 'miracle' was being explained to the youngest class. 'If you prayed that your teacher would have a cold and be absent the next morning, and if that actually happened, what would that seem to be?' I asked. 'A coincidence', was the reply.

'Which number is higher, one or ten?' The 8-year-old boy considered my question carefully. 'One. Would you like me to prove it?' I nodded, curious 'Well, in spelling class we write the numbers down the page starting with one at the top and ten down at the bottom. One is always higher up the page.' He was quite serious.

Children with specific learning difficulties can often adopt failure or a poor standard of performance as an intentional strategy. If they choose to present themselves as a non-achiever rather than as an underachiever, little will be demanded of them. It is less demoralizing for them to set consistently low standards for themselves than to disappoint parents and teachers who have high expectations.

Maurice (11)

Maurice wrote the classically dreary weekend diary. No risk taking for him. 'I got up. I had breakfast. I went to the shops. I had lunch. I played football. I watched TV. I had supper. I went to bed.' He was asked if he had been as bored writing this as I had been reading it. I talked about 'attention grabbers', opening sentences which startled the reader and tempted him to read on. 'I want something to amaze me in my tray on Monday,' I told him. His offering duly arrived. 'My gun was still smoking after I had shot all the teachers,' it began.

DEPENDENCY

'Learned failure' is a not uncommon description of the 'can't try, won't try, don't know how to begin' attitude adopted as a defence mechanism. 'Learned inadequacy' could be a term coined to describe the acceptance by some dyslexic children that their performance will naturally be below standard. This attitude is often fostered by well-intentioned adults. A child who is dyslexic needs more, not less, practice in survival skills if they are to keep their self-esteem intact. Competence in the day-to-day skills of answering the telephone, shopping, ordering a meal in a cafe or planning a journey are all part and parcel of a broader education, whether this is provided at school or at home. To imply to a child that they are dyslexic and therefore incompetent or in need of special protection is probably the most damaging approach which can be adopted.

Nancy (10), Ben (11) and Martin (12)

I asked Nancy's father if she was allowed to cook at home. 'But of course,' he replied. 'She makes the toast for breakfast.' Could she not, I enquired, be promoted to scrambled eggs or even scones? Ben's mother told me firmly that he 'could not be trusted to carry a plate of biscuits through to the sitting room'. Another boy, Martin, who was slightly older than Ben, had never made a public telephone call or taken the bus or Underground by himself. He was unsure of the value of money. He was not really safe alone on the road, since he was transported everywhere by car. Yet he was within measurable distance of entering his teens, where parental ties must be stretched or even broken. His siblings, both older and younger, were allowed much more freedom.

In academic matters, dyslexic children will often have become dependent on help and support from teachers and their parents during their early years in a mainstream school. Without it they could not have survived. In the long run, if allowed to continue, this dependency breeds hostility, self-denigration and apathy in the classroom. To halt the downward spiral, in a specialist school children should be taught self-monitoring and coping strategies and should be encouraged to take risks without fear of ridicule. Failure in controlled circumstances, if followed up by the immediate teaching of preventive strategies, can be therapeutic but must lead to clearer insight and alternative, more successful approaches.

ENHANCING CHILDREN'S SELF-ESTEEM

Building confidence is partly a matter of public image. This can be enhanced by creating specific roles with genuine responsibility within the school. Prefects can be selected following guidelines which are fully understood by the children themselves. They must be polite, well behaved and kind to others. They must be good ambassadors for the school. In this context, with careful preparation and training, they often greatly enjoy taking visitors on tours. Monitors can be drawn from the younger groups and be given specific tasks which give them status in particular areas such as games, sport, music or computers. Class captains may be usefully assigned jobs within the classroom, adapted to take account of age and maturity. All the groups can have a forum for discussion at a weekly meeting. Suggestions, requests or complaints can be submitted to the Headteacher or to a full staff meeting and will be seriously considered. Many of these dyslexic office-holders would not have sported any badge of merit in a conventional school, where their perceived inadequacies would have precluded them from selection.

A good forum for the acknowledgement of success is a full weekly assembly where children can be formally and publicly praised for academic achievement, for acts of efficiency or kindness, for being considerate or for showing initiative, indeed for excellence manifested in any area. They can exhibit their models, paintings or projects. They can receive formal certificates to put on their walls at home proclaiming that they have been promoted from pencil to pen or completed a touch-typing programme successfully. Public recognition and acknowledgement are welcome, whether it be the genuine fascination of all present when a complicated electric circuit is switched on and a light bulb flashes or the wholehearted clapping which greets a noisy but musical performance on the drums or sympathetic admiration when a younger child demonstrates a newly acquired mastery of the art of skipping. As the children grow in self-respect and confidence, they become noticeably more generous in applauding the triumphs of others. Negative feelings of failure produce snide remarks, envious denial of peer achievement and the short, sharp retaliatory foray in the cloakroom or on the stairs. The answer is to ensure that every child has some area of prowess or originality which can be publicly proclaimed. Such initiatives as writing a letter to the Queen, bringing in grandfather's war medals or cleaning out the class goldfish tank can all be suitably commended. There is always something to praise.

Showing children how to boost the morale of others can be an excellent way of enhancing self-respect. Older children enjoy visiting younger children in their classrooms and either reading to them or listening to their hesitant attempts to decode a simple text. The older children become aware of how far they themselves have progressed and look back more objectively and with greater satisfaction at the problems they have overcome. The admiration and respect of the younger children increases older pupils' confidence. An unexpected outcome can be the fostering of the protective instinct in the older children and a reduction in the teasing or even bullying that is so difficult to eradicate in any school, even with constant staff supervision.

SOCIAL PROBLEMS

It would indeed be naive to assume that teasing and bullying can be entirely eliminated, especially in a school where many of the children have been victims in the past and either continue to invite attack or, on becoming more confident, are transformed into the aggressors. Teaching the victim evasive or self-assertive tactics is usually as successful in the short term as persuading the aggressor to modify their behaviour. In the long term some of the children who initially show less tolerance and sympathy with their weaker brethren develop remarkable insight later on when they are given responsibility and feel more assured about their own status and standing.

It is not uncommon for dyslexic children to have social problems. Their lack of friends, the apparent contempt of their classmates, their failure to respond appropriately to adults and their proneness to confrontation with parents and teachers are all factors which undermine self-esteem and distort the child's perception of their identity and capabilities. The more these children are viewed holistically, the more apparent it becomes that these problems are not the emotional by-product of dyslexia but a part of its very nature. It is hard for anyone searching the mind for a fact, figure or proper name to retain eye contact with a listener. How much more embarrassing for dyslexic children, who are frequently searching their memories for the right word or phrase. Losing eye contact, they miss other clues and ignore facial expression, body language and tone of voice. Formulating with difficulty their own responses, they fail to register how the conversation is developing and repeat what others have just said or do not realize that the topic has been abandoned. Whether it is in class, with a group of children in the playground or sitting round the television with the family, their utterances may appear at best quaint but at worst tactless and even provocative. Rebuff or rebuke will be taken as a personal insult and will arouse a strongly negative response in the dyslexic child, with possible tantrums or stormy protests, which may seem out of all proportion to the nature of the incident. Deep at the root of the problem is the conviction of dyslexic children that their treatment is 'not fair', that they are being misunderstood, discriminated against, undervalued or victimized. It is for this reason that any code of discipline must be clearly spelled out to these children.

DISCIPLINE

It seems logical to assume that the dyslexic, with poor sequencing skills and with established difficulties in verbalizing their thought processes, does not work out in advance the simple practicalities of cause and effect. Especially if there is any degree of hyperactivity, these children are likely to be impulsive (for this reason, incidentally, they are often accident-prone). They will almost inevitably create trouble for themselves at school and at home by acting without envisaging the consequences or even recognizing the direct link between what they have done and the reaction of adults or their peers. Intent on showing their drawing to the teacher, they career across the classroom, knocking into other pupils' desks, demanding immediate attention. In a sudden burst of anger at an ill-timed remark in the playground, they fling out an arm and make disastrous contact with the front teeth of an opponent. Unexpectedly identifying their mother on the other side of the street they may scamper across without stopping to look out for oncoming traffic. They will irritatingly answer questions out of turn in class, talk when they are asked to be silent in assembly or appear wilfully to ignore instructions on the games field.

Such actions are often not deliberate but appear to be so. They invite rebuke and, in fact, for the smooth running of the school, the culprit must be reprimanded. 'I got told off', 'I got an order mark', 'I got sent out of the room', the children will protest, 'and I don't know why'. Their misconduct has been explained to them and they know the rules but when it comes to applying them, they fail to make the proper connections or draw the correct conclusions and therefore sanctions are fiercely resented.

The idea that dyslexics should be exonerated from blame just because they are dyslexic is foolish and even dangerous. They will have to comply in real life with the rules and regulations of the community and, as adults, with the law itself. The answer must be to teach these children to exert self-discipline and self-regulation, rather than imposing a strict code of behaviour, which they will not internalize or remember, through punishment or withdrawal of privilege. If this is not done, dyslexic children will be harder to place in a mainstream school, as misconduct compounds learning difficulties. Another important consideration is that when pupils are disciplined for any misdemeanour, they almost invariably become resentful and preoccupied for the rest of the day or even longer and valuable learning time is wasted.

The aim is neither to restrain nor protect them, but to teach them social awareness, consideration for others, insight into their own feelings and those of other people, self-control and strategies for staying out of trouble. It is worth noting that since dyslexics are often unpredictable themselves in their responses, it is harder for them to foresee how others will react. Teaching them to be effective 'people watchers' and encouraging parents to explain to their children how to gauge the consequences of a certain pattern of events or course of action can be helpful. This may prevent these children from inadvertently upsetting or annoying both adults and their peers.

Anna (9)

Anna had such arguments with her mother every morning, often over quite trivial matters, that she was usually still fuming and furious when she arrived at school. Her mood of anger and irritation was almost tangible and she could remain sulky and rude for much of the rest of the school day. During a long discussion together over a sandwich lunch (a pleasant alternative to a more formal interview), ways were suggested in which she could transform the morning encounters with her mother through a couple of well-directed complimentary remarks, backed up with such helpful actions as having her school bag ready by the front door or leaving her room reasonably tidy. This, I explained to Anna, would enable her to be in charge of the situation. She would be the one to avert confrontation and to initiate friendly overtures. It would restore to her, hopefully, the feeling that she was in control. Anna decided to try it out. To my delight she seemed much more relaxed in the mornings.

Two weeks later I caught her leaping down the stairs four steps at a time. I was particularly annoyed because I had been talking to all the children about the dangers inherent in this sort of behaviour. Someone could get hurt. She preempted anything further I could say by catching my eye, smiling warmly and remarking, 'That was such a lovely prayer you read us in assembly this morning. My favourite, actually'. I was stopped in my tracks. Anna had learnt a lesson about deflecting wrath.

SELF-MONITORING SKILLS

Few children will catch on as quickly as Anna to the skills of manipulating the response of others through the modification of their own behaviour. A weekly 'Club', run by the Occupational Therapist and Speech and Language Therapist, can target children who have difficulties responding appropriately to adults or their peers and, in a small group, teach them to identify and evaluate the responses of others. Just as importantly, they can learn to see their own behaviour in a more objective light.

ROLE PLAY

Often, with dyslexic children, it is emotional reaction that is at the root of their misconduct. If properly handled, small group discussions after an 'incident' in the playground or the classroom can defuse situations. The 'culprit' and 'victim' appraise the event with one or two of their most sensible peers, who act as witnesses. The Headteacher's part in the proceedings is to encourage the children to take the initiative in these discussions and to create an atmosphere where the truth can be revealed without eliciting an unduly censorious or angry response. Role play can help to achieve greater objectivity, often through imagining a parallel case to the one under discussion and allowing the 'culprit' to play the part of the judge and to explain why some conduct is unacceptable and how it can be prevented. Often children will be more critical of their own conduct in giving judgement than an adult would dare to be. With the older children, a parallel case can be drawn from an imaginary workplace scenario to attain better insight and an added feeling of importance.

Joseph (12)
'You are grown up, and you have established a successful garage business. You discover that one of your employees has played a practical joke on the others by switching the labels on the equipment. Lives could have been in danger. What would you do? 'Fire him,' was the immediate reply. A healthy discussion grew out of these comments. Sympathetic peer pressure can be therapeutic.

SANCTIONS

Opportunities can be created during the school week when the code of discipline can be discussed with the children. The Headteacher can take an assembly which the staff do not attend. This is a good chance to explain and rationalize the school rules to the children with questions from the floor encouraged. Such discussions can also be initiated in lessons with individual classes.

Anthony (12)
It was Anthony, a senior pupil, who had a good idea in response to the frequent complaint of 'It's not fair', that a system of cards should be devised, echoing the sanctions on the football field. After any serious breach of the rules a card would be given to the child, stating exactly why it had been issued.

It is important that the child's parents should be kept informed of any problems on a regular routine basis, as it is not helpful if first indications of trouble only appear in the end-of-term report. The children themselves should be encouraged to identify patterns of misconduct. Is it poor behaviour in unstructured situations, such as lunchtime or playtime, which is the problem? Has the child been constantly disrupting lessons, teasing younger children or brawling in the cloakrooms? Is it one lesson or one teacher or one area of the school day which is creating friction or is it a particular pupil who regularly causes the child to overstep the bounds of acceptable behaviour? It becomes much easier to discuss solutions if root causes are clearly recognized.

AVOIDANCE STRATEGIES

The strategies which children adopt to enable them to avoid those areas of the curriculum which they find hardest or most uncongenial must be tactfully diverted.

John (9)

John was brought to the office with clockwork regularity whenever there was a spelling test. His face would be ashen white and he would be clutching his stomach and claiming to feel sick. If his bluff was called and he was sent back to the classroom, he might indeed throw up his breakfast. If it was accepted that he was genuinely unwell and he was sent home, another day was wasted.

One morning I simply said to him, as he lay there limp and listless, 'John, I feel I need a break. I'm going out shopping. Would you like to come too? He rose without a word, his acute stomach ache forgotten or vanished, and trotted beside me down the road. I gave him some money to choose a book for his classroom and he spent an inordinate amount of time selecting a book of jokes which were just not bawdy enough to incur my censure. He went back to the classroom on our return without any fuss. Subsequently spelling tests appeared to become more tolerable and he did not return to the sickbay on a regular basis.

POSITIVE REINFORCEMENT

Remedial education is not just a matter of helping the child to acquire basic academic skills. If dyslexic children can be taught to tolerate lessons, people or situations they dislike, they can acquire a positive advantage. Most importantly, these children need to develop the ability to verbalize and communicate their opinions and their feelings. Violent reaction may be unnecessary if they can explain their problems coherently. Insight into how to control the potentially explosive situation creates confidence. The reaction of others is reassuringly positive when the child becomes more amenable and less disconcertingly impulsive.

They now feel better able to exercise self-discipline and to exert a more determining influence on their own record of behaviour.

Positive reinforcement, red marks, star badges, warmly appreciative comments when the child acts sensibly and considerably, all these are encouraging proof to children that they are successfully earning the respect and admiration of those around them. It can be assumed that most children of primary school age normally want to please, unless they have been antagonized. Showing a dyslexic child how to do so should be a priority.

Conclusion

> *Ken (24)*
> A letter came from Ken, a former pupil. 'Without you,' he wrote, 'I would not be where I am now.' Flattering though this seemed at first glance, closer inspection revealed that the individual concerned was in Timbuktu. Was that where he wanted to be? Had he taken a wrong turning? He himself conveyed a note of faint astonishment in his letter. Ken, in fact, had joined the army, which had been his childhood dream, and was on desert manoeuvres. If he had not acquired the necessary literacy and numeracy skills to pass his examinations, he would never have made a career in the army or achieved at a level commensurate with his true ability.

Enabling the child to be an independent learner, establishing basic academic skills and instilling confidence must be the important targets for all those involved with these children. The Headteacher has the task of orchestrating the contributions of the professionals, pupils and parents to achieve solutions.

There must be clear vision, identified aims and determination that goals will be achieved. Above all, the Headteacher must inspire the confidence, enthusiasm and self-esteem of all concerned to help to break down barriers and release the full potential of the dyslexic child.

References

Chasty, H. and Friel, J. (1995) *Children with Special Needs. Assessment, Law and Practice. Caught in the Act,* 3rd edn, Jessica Kingsley, London.

Gardner, H. (1983) *Frames of Mind. The Theory of Multiple Intelligences*, Basic Books, New York.

Hornsby, B. (1984) *Overcoming Dyslexia*, Martin Dunitz Ltd, London.

Milne, A.A. (1924) *When We were Very Young*, Methuen, and Co. Ltd, London.

Orton, C. (1994), The 1993 Education Act. *Dyslexia Contact*, 13(2), 8–9.

Ostler, C. (1991) *A Parents' Survival Guide*, Ammonite Books, Godalming.

Russell, P. (1994) The Code of Practice: new partnerships for children with special educational needs. *British Journal of Special Education*, 21(2), 48–52.

West, T. (1991) *In the Mind's Eye*, Prometheus, New York.

11 *Conclusion*

Peter Gilchrist

The dyslexic syndrome that we have discussed throughout this book is clearly of considerable complexity in theoretical terms, diagnosis and prescription of treatment. We are now well aware that the condition embraces the processing of letter symbols, whether decoding and reading or encoding and spelling and producing written language. It also embraces the much more complex world of sophisticated information processing, whose influence is frequently found in later adolescence as children struggle to cope with formal examinations. There are also many other complex issues that may profoundly affect a dyslexic child's performance or capacity to respond to treatment. The management of dyslexia is seldom, if ever, straightforward. Fairley House has gathered together a team of experts, all of whom have a significant contribution to make in the diagnosis and assessment of dyslexia, as well as its later management.

Throughout the book, each specialist has opened a door into their own particular department, shown us their areas of expertise and allowed us to develop an understanding of how they perceive specific learning disabilities and how they feel they can most usefully contribute. It is appropriate that each should have their own viewpoint and perception of the children with whom they work, but what is equally clear is that they see themselves as part of an integrated team, each member of which is making a major contribution.

Much time has been spent in surveying the variety of specialists who deal with the lives of children with specific learning disabilities. Even for the authors and the practitioners themselves this has drawn together their feelings and philosophies as far as the condition and its management is concerned. It has certainly highlighted very clearly that we are discussing an interdependent programme. Without the availability and possible involvement of the entire team, diagnosis and treatment may never be quite complete.

So often the multidisciplinary approach to specific learning disabilities implies hurried assessment, a class teacher with more than 30 children to manage, intermittent visits from a remedial teacher and the support of the rest of the team if and when they prove available. It is a great privilege to work as part of so complex a wheel, the spokes of which are complete.

I felt that to clarify our thinking and emphasize how the involvement of the entire team may prove absolutely essential, we should work through a final case study.

Susan (7 years and 8 months)

When Susan presented herself to Fairley House she was a little over 7½ years of age, living in north London, with a mother and father who travelled a great deal on business and a brother and sister, both older than herself, who went to local secondary schools. David, her older brother, had specific learning disabilities in his primary school days and these had been given a modicum of support and he seemed to be coping adequately, although his school reports were always poor.

Susan's problem had come forcibly to the attention of her class teacher when she began to notice, increasingly, that Susan was often in a daydream and seemed to have lost contact with what was going on around her. When this feature of her behaviour was drawn to her parents' attention they looked further and found that, for a child of her age, she had made little or no start with reading, spelling or written work and that even her mathematics were a year behind her chronological age. Doubts were expressed as to her overall intellectual ability, but her parents felt that she was at least average and that there were spikes of ability that seemed to suggest that she might be very much brighter than this.

However, late-developing language – she was at least four before she began to speak effectively at all – had left its legacy in her early school years, making her sound rather slow and unresponsive. Even at the point of her assessment, her vocabulary was limited and her ability to express herself far from mature. She was desperately easily muddled by incoming language, especially complex instructions.

In discussion with Susan's mother, it became apparent that after a rather difficult birth, Susan had come home from hospital and although physical development had passed by relatively normally, she had always been very inclined to colds, was very adenoidal and given to constant bouts of otitis media (ear infections). She began nursery school at three, but was constantly away with very unpleasant bouts of tonsillitis, which also involved further infections of her ears. This not only interrupted the early stages of her schooling, but left her feeling tired and lethargic. Eventually, at 4½ she had an ear, nose and throat investigation and it was decided to remove her tonsils and adenoids and to fit grommet tubes to help her hearing.

Susan started more formal schooling shortly after her fifth birthday and was very unhappy and restless at the outset, with constant floods of tears leaving her mother in the mornings. She seemed to be a rather sad, remote little girl, very given to emotional outbursts, especially if a teacher became cross. Progress was minimal. By her second year she was clearly falling further and further behind her peers and, to make matters worse, her older brother David was becoming increasingly difficult and there were threats that he might have to be taken into the care of the local authority, as he kept running away and being extremely rude and abusive to the entire family. On one desperately unpleasant evening he returned home, having been drinking beer with his friends – very much under age – had a fight with his mother, hit her and knocked her down, cutting her head. This led to his being taken into care for some six weeks, after which he seemed to be a little more stable.

By the time the assessment at Fairley House arose, it was quite clear that Susan would need considerable understanding and support if she was to begin to bridge the gap between her potential and the academic skills of her peers. Her inability to cope in class was becoming more and more painful, isolating her still further.

She was also a rather disorganized little girl, who never seemed to arrive in time for lessons and was always losing vital equipment. Her mother reported that her bedroom at home was chaotic and it was a wonder that Susan could ever find the things that she needed. This was made worse by her very evident naivety and tendency to rush in where 'angels fear to tread', only to be distressed by the very clear disruption that she so often caused by doing so. She was a bewildered, unhappy, failing little girl. Her parents, who were under great emotional pressure from their son, were now shattered to find that they had a further problem to face within the family. It might be helpful to piece together the valuable contribution which each member of the team would make to Susan's welfare.

It is important that after courage has been summoned up to make an initial phone call to a school like Fairley House, the reception is kind, gentle, friendly and informative. It was therefore crucial that early bridges were built between Susan's parents and the school and an understanding of the syndrome, its implications and possible treatment are made clear.

Both the **Headteacher** and her support staff have a very considerable role to play. Quite understandably, an upset or panicked parent may simply not return for further investigation and Susan would have to continue in the bewildering world of specific learning disabilities. Furthermore, at this particular stage in the process, the other members of the team have not yet been invited to become involved, so they have no contribution to make.

However, if we assume that a rapport was beginning to be built up and an initial appointment was made, we can then look at some of the early answers that we hoped to achieve during the morning of Susan's initial assessment.

From the initial interview and the family questionnaire, we knew Susan's sex and age. We knew that her parents were together, but that her father travelled and was often absent from the family home; we knew that there were two older children, one of whom had a learning difficulty and sounded severely maladjusted. This added considerable emotional weight to the problems of the family. Susan's auditory processing had almost certainly been impaired by her ear, nose and throat history and she herself had become thoroughly demoralized. Staff in her present school questioned Susan's overall ability and appeared to be suggesting that poor performance was simply an indication of her limited intellectual capacity.

It followed that one of the first questions that we needed to answer was 'Exactly how bright is Susan?' Psychometric evaluation with the **Educational Psychologist** should certainly reveal this information. Her intelligence proved to be high average. It also emerged at this stage that she had difficulties with the organization and processing of language, poor short-term memory function, both auditory and visual, slow and awkward fine motor coordination and difficulties of spatial awareness and visual perception. She was crosslateral (with a dominant right hand but left eye) and her reading, spelling and mathematics were all retarded. In the case of her reading, this was almost two years below her chronological age and her comprehension was poor, even at this rather primitive stage of reading.

We were already coming to know rather more about this little girl and, at this stage in the diagnosis, it was important that her language processing difficulties, both diagnostically and in terms of prescribing treatment, were looked at in considerable detail by the **Speech and**

Language Therapist. She was able to determine to what extent Susan's problems were a residual issue, resulting from her early tonsil, adenoid and otitis media difficulties which in themselves had been quite severe, requiring considerable treatment, and to what extent a further language processing disorder was involved.

The decision was made that she did not have articulation defects and that her poor communication skills were the result of a mild deficit in the processing of spoken language, which resulted in the late development of language in the first place, compounded by her ear, nose and throat history. It was felt that this would take at least two sessions a week, one individual and one small group, together with support and liaison with the class teacher. The Speech and Language Therapist also noticed the rather dreamy, momentary absences from which Susan suffered and which were further disrupting her processing.

The problems of fine motor coordination and visual perception which had begun to emerge from the Educational Psychologist's investigations were then looked at in far greater detail by the **Occupational Therapist**. She was able to determine that there was, indeed, a mild degree of dyspraxia and that Susan would require a programme of sensory integration to deal with this problem, together with considerable work on her balance, body posture, pencil hold and letter formation.

Susan's day in Fairley House was completed by a visit to the Headteacher, where the approach was no longer as structured and intellectually demanding as it had been for the rest of her time. She found this session much more fun and more relaxing. Not only did this finish her day on a pleasant and cheerful note, but it allowed the Headteacher to see a little girl in action, about whom she knew a great deal from the case conference that had been conducted following the specialist sessions. She was able to look at teachability, capacity to respond, level of enthusiasm, level of motivation and so forth. Indeed, it would now be her responsibility to decide whether or not Susan would truly benefit from time in Fairley House School, using her own observations and those of the specialists as the basis for this decision, together with the wishes and aspirations of the family.

In the consultation that followed with the parents and the Educational Psychologist, Susan's 'absences' were discussed yet again and the possibility that this might have been a petit mal type of absence seizure was discussed. It was clearly very important, not only for the child's health but for her education, that she maintained her concentration and did not have her processing continually interrupted in this way.

As is so often the case with dyslexic children, it also appeared that Susan had not established a reference eye at this point in her development and this too might have been hindering her progress. Indeed, towards the end of her time she fidgeted constantly, rubbing her eyes, and this seemed to hinder her concentration still further.

The school suggested that this problems should be investigated through the family doctor. The need for a referral to the **Paediatrician** was now quite clear. There was certainly nobody else in the team competent to make a firm diagnosis of petit mal. Equally, he was the specialist who could prescribe medication and this would then be linked through the family's general practitioner. As matters emerged, the Paediatrician found no evidence of petit mal, which was a great relief to Susan's family, but he did feel that she was experiencing a mild degree of attention deficit disorder. He did not consider that this required treatment or medication at that particular point. He felt sure that this problem had been exacerbated by a visual anomaly, to which the Headteacher alluded when she observed the anguished rubbing of the eyes and increasing distractibility that were a part of Susan's problems in the latter part of the morning at Fairley House.

Ann Wilson, the **Orthoptist**, has described cases not dissimilar to Susan in the chapter describing her work. Susan did indeed present very considerable problems in this area, including lack of a reference eye, and the advice of the Orthoptist proved invaluable, both diagnostically and in designing appropriate remediation. Her diagnostic conclusion was that Susan was experiencing an intermittent divergent squint. Early in the day she appeared perfectly normal, but as she began to tire so she lost control of the squint and one eye wandered outwards so that she looked as if she was not paying attention. Susan's problems were further exacerbated by acquired myopia, which made her distance vision blurred. It was hardly surprising that she 'switched off' and her eyes became itchy and tired! Glasses and a minor operation made a radical difference.

A place was offered to Susan and gladly accepted. She arrived early the following September in some trepidation, but quickly found both the children and teachers accepting and warm. By the end of the first morning she had settled in remarkably happily.

A great deal of time was spent over those first few weeks settling Susan into her class and helping her to realize that the failures of the past need not continue into the future. It was vital that she began to see that each day would present her with hurdles marginally higher than those that she had ever cleared before, but always within her capabilities. Confidence, a willingness and capacity to take risks and to 'have a go' were all a vital part of these early weeks in encouraging Susan to be 'available for learning'.

The **class teachers**, Nick Rees and Angela Dominy, have described in their chapter the process through which a child goes in order to acquire adequate phonic skills, written literacy skills, numeracy skills and so forth. Their work is supported on an individual and small group basis by the specialist **remedial teachers**, who in Susan's case looked particularly at her phonic weaknesses and poor auditory processing.

The Speech and Language Therapists also played a part in Susan's management, especially in her capacity to organize and process spoken language. it was, after all, unrealistic to expect her to process effective written language if she could neither think nor say it. Her dyspraxic problems, necessitating a programme of sensory integration, needed regular management by the Occupational Therapist. Hence, class support in a medium-sized group of 12 children, adhering as closely as realistically possible to the National Curriculum, together with specialist support, all became a carefully integrated part of the process.

Finally, we must reflect back to the other sources of unhappiness in Susan's family. He brother, David, had been taken into care, her father was away on ever longer trips and her mother was becoming increasingly distraught. With the best will in the world, specialist staff in the school were unable to provide help in depth for Susan's mother or to enable Susan herself to understand how the world around her worked and how she must relate to it if she was to be happy and effective. Fortunately, Fairley House has the support and help of a **Counsellor** and she too now played a vital role.

Gradually, these various threads were drawn together. Susan's family was supported and she herself began to feel more secure and her progress developed socially, emotionally and academically. In due course, and this took 3 years, the smile returned, her posture was more composed and confident, school work progressed on a happily upward curve. Susan looked and sounded altogether different and was now ready to move back into the mainstream of education to face the very considerable challenges of secondary schooling and public examinations in due course.

If we reflect for a final moment on Susan and her complex dilemma, it is impossible to see how her problems could have been adequately diagnosed or her treatment effectively managed had it not been for the full, integrated and sensitive support of a considerable team of specialists. The effective management of specific learning disabilities does and must always revolve around the team.

Conclusion

From the chapters written by the various specialists in Fairley House we gather a depth of insight into their work, both diagnostic and therapeutic, much of which is alluded to in this conclusion. However, in the day-to-day life of a busy school like Fairley House, each specialist anticipates the support of the remainder of the team in reaching a full and detailed understanding of the child, the problems, possible treatment regimes and therefore what their own personal contribution might be.

If we look back over the management of Susan and her rather complex dilemma, it is perhaps worth speculating as to which of these specialists could have been withdrawn from the team with no detriment to Susan and her welfare. As her case moved in turn from the initial information gathering of the family questionnaire, through the gentle, professional interviewing of the Headteacher to the full and detailed diagnostic process, it is quite clear that Susan's management would have been seriously disadvantaged had we been unable to involve all the various specialists. There will always, of course, be cases which do not need to utilize the entire team, but its availability is vital.

Furthermore, problems may arise during the two or three-year treatment process in Fairley House and these will need to be investigated at this point in the child's development.

Where children are being taught outside the environment of a specialist school an awareness of what is available within each of these specialisms is crucial for parents, specialist remedial teachers and other professionals who may become involved. It allows them to make appropriate onward referral to the specialists in their area if this proves necessary.

Without a sophisticated understanding of the problem in itself, the various guises in which it may come and the contribution that a complex team can make, it is difficult for treatment to move beyond the relatively superficial.

Glossary

Accommodation Normally refers to physical or psychological adjustment in preparation for an incoming stimulus or change of stimulus. When referring to vision it applies to the adjustment of the shape of the lens of the eye to compensate for the distance of the object of focus from the retina.

Aphasia Refers to a profound speech disorder which has a radical impact on the individual's capacity to organize and process incoming language and often to produce effective speech. It is generally presumed that aphasia is due to lesions in both Broca's and Wernicke's areas of the brain.

Asperger's syndrome This is best understood as a mild form of autism, demonstrating itself in inappropriate behaviour and emotional responses and a considerable naivety in an individual's capacity to interpret the feelings and body language of those around them. The majority of Asperger's individuals can be helped to adjust, at least to some extent, to relatively normal social interactions.

Associative Usually any learned, functional connection between two or more elements.

Attention deficit disorder (with or without hyperactivity) Characterized by individuals who cannot remain on task for more than a relatively brief period of time, who are largely incapable of coping with selective attention in that they are as distracted by redundant stimuli around them as they are by the task in hand. Their social responses are naive, disinhibited and, at times, inappropriate. Those experiencing hyperactivity will find themselves constantly on the move, fidgeting restlessly as they struggle to process information.

Auditory acuity The ability to hear sound, sharpness of hearing.

Auditory perception   The identification, organization and interpretation of information through the ears, subdivided as follows:

Attention – the ability to know when to respond to sounds

Blending – the ability to blend together separate speech sounds to form words

Discrimination – the ability to distinguish between sounds and/or noises, e.g. between a car or lorry or individual speech sounds

Figure–ground – selecting specific sounds from an environment of many, e.g. picking out teacher's voice in a noisy classroom

Localization – the ability to recognize the source/direction of a sound

Memory – the storage of auditorally presented information long enough to analyse it

Sequencing – reproduction of the correct order of sounds/information.

Balance   The body's ability to maintain an upright posture against gravity.

Static balance – the ability to keep a stationary position through coordination of muscle activity in counteracting an opposing force, e.g. when pushed

Dynamic balance – the ability to maintain an upright posture while the body is moving, e.g. running to catch a ball.

Binocular function   Describes the ability to use two eyes as a pair to produce a single visual image.

Body image   Awareness of one's own body and its orientation, position and movement in space.

Cerebral   Pertaining to the brain.

Cerebral dominance   The leading hemisphere, right or left, of the brain which appears to determine an individual's hand, eye, foot, etc. preference. See also *laterality, hemisphere.*

Choreiform movement   Non-repetitive, dancelike movements with a random, irregular quality.

Chromosome   A microscopic body in the nucleus of a cell which is conspicuous during mitosis. Chromosomes carry the genes, the basic hereditary units. Each species has a constant, normal number of chromosomes. For example, there are 46 in human somatic cells arranged in 23 pairs. The term literally means 'coloured body' and chromosomes were so named because they stain deeply with basic dyes.

Closure   The ability to recognize a whole when one or more parts are missing. This applies especially to the auditory, visual (see also visual perception) and tactile senses.

Cloze procedure A testing technique. Words or parts of words are omitted for the child to supply or complete. It is used to assess or teach grammatical or semantic competence.

Cognitive Describing intellectual activity, knowing as opposed to feeling.

Concept An idea, abstract or concrete, mentally established through interpretation of experiences and usually embodied in a word, e.g. a young child learning 'hot' by association with fire, cooker, sun, etc. All language is built up this way.

Consistency The essential notion that a test will produce the same result when administered repeatedly under similar conditions.

Coordination Combination of different bodily actions to perform a functional task.

Bilateral coordination – coordination of both sides of the body simultaneously, e.g. catching a large ball, where both hands work together, or writing, where one hand writes while the other supports the paper
Gross motor coordination – coordination of muscle activity to carry out large movement patterns, e.g. running, walking, hopping, jumping
Fine motor coordination – coordination of small muscle groups for functional tasks involving precision and small movements, e.g. finger movements when writing
Visual–motor coordination – the ability to focus on the visual aspect of a task whilst carrying out the motor activities needed simultaneously, e.g. catching a ball involves hand–eye coordination and kicking a ball involves foot–eye coordination.

Correlation The relationship between two sets of test scores. In statistics a perfect relationship gives a correlation of +1.0, complete lack of relationship is 0 and the exact opposite is –1.0.

Crosslaterality See *laterality*.

Digraphs Two letters, vowels or consonants, which combine to make a single sound, e.g. th, sh, ar, aw, ee.

Directionality Internal awareness of direction, i.e. the ability to orientate oneself within space.

Discrimination The ability to perceive differences between two or more stimuli.

Dysarthria A general term for defective speaking, impaired articulatory ability. Typically used to refer to cases resulting from peripheral motor or muscular defects.

Dyscalculia　A specific difficulty with mathematical functions.

Dysgraphia　Difficulty with mechanical aspects of writing, i.e. poor letter formation and presentation of written work.

Dysphasia　This implies a comparative disability in the capacity to process spoken language and to organize incoming language, frequently demonstrated in an incapacity to understand complex instructions or in inappropriate and at times even bizarre spoken responses.

Dyspraxia　Fundamentally, a difficulty in interpreting verbal signals in motor terms. It implies a lack of effective sensory integration, poor spatial organization and motor planning. Individuals can appear awkward, clumsy and, in general terms, thoroughly disorganized.

Echolalia　Meaningless repetition of words or phrases just spoken by another person.

Emmetropia　Normal vision, in the sense that when the eye is at rest the light is refracted so that the focus is directly on the retina.

Encoding　The process of changing one form of symbol into another, as in transferring the spoken word into the relevant written form in spelling/writing.

Flash cards　Letters, words or sentences placed upon cards which are briefly exposed to the child as a teaching technique to encourage speedy word recognition.

Graded reading scheme　A series of books arranged according to difficulty.

Grapheme　A written symbol representing a speech sound (*phoneme*).

Handedness　The preferred hand which may differ for different activities or may be different from the preferred eye, ear or foot. See *laterality*.

Hemisphere　One of the two halves, left and right, of the brain. The left hemisphere controls the motor activity of the right side of the body, the right hemisphere controls the left of the body. Many human activities require a preferred limb or organ, e.g. for writing, kicking, playing tennis, using a camera. In these instances one of the hemispheres is said to have *cerebral dominance*. Some functions are specialized in one or other hemisphere, e.g. the speech and language centres are normally in the left hemisphere, while appreciation of rhythm and music is specific to the right hemisphere.

Holistic　Looking at a subject in its entirety and not just at its constituent parts.

Hyperactivity Excessive and often uncontrolled body movements or general activity.

Hypoactivity Below normal levels of physical activity, listless behaviour.

Hysterical This must be clearly differentiated from the popular image of the hysterical, out of control, weeping individual. Hysterical blindness, for example, will deprive the patient of effective vision and yet there will be no apparent organic causation. There are well-recorded cases of hysterical paralysis, including hysterical ataxia, as well as hysterical deafness. The condition tends to be associated with a personality type but the symptoms are very real as far as the patient is concerned and may be totally disabling, but treatment will be directed more at stress and anxiety management than any organic disorder.

Ideation The formation or relation of ideas prior to beginning a task or action.

Kinaesthetic Perception obtained through muscle awareness and movement. Feedback to brain from muscle receptors in limbs and body when a movement is made.

Laterality Pertaining to the left and right sides of the body. Mixed or crosslaterality refers to mixed left or right side preference for certain activities, e.g. dominant right hand combined with dominant left eye.

Metacognition An understanding of the learning process and an awareness of how it can be analysed, developed and controlled through discovering how to crossreference and draw logical conclusions.

Maturation lag A delay in certain aspects of physical development.

Modality The pathways by which the individual receives information and thereby learns. The 'modality concept' suggests that some individuals learn better through one modality than another. For instance, a child may process information more efficiently through their visual modality, perhaps learning sight words by tracing methods, rather than through auditory, phonic methods.

Morpheme The smallest meaning-bearing unit in the language, which can be a single concept, word, root, prefix or suffix.

Motor movement

Fine motor – activities involving small areas of the musculature of the body, e.g. writing, cutting

Gross motor – activities involving large areas of the musculature of the body and particularly the large muscle groups, e.g. skipping

Motor perceptual – this describes the linkage between the child's brain and their body's capacity to respond physically to the environment.

Multidisciplinary   Implies the involvement of several different disciplines, often professions, in the resolution of problems.

Multisensory   Using all the pathways – visual, auditory, kinaesthetic – simultaneously, with particular reference to teaching methods with dyslexic children.

Occlusion   Means fundamentally an obstruction, a block, a closure. In the case of dyslexic children it normally refers to the patching of one eye to allow for the strengthening of the other.

Ocular   Pertaining to the eye.

Olfactory   Pertaining to the sense of smell or act of smelling.

Orientation   The chosen direction, in English from left to right, of reading along a line of print. It can also refer to the direction of letters, where reversals and confusions may exist, e.g. m/w; h/y; b/d. It may also refer to the child's personal orientation in space, for example, their capacity to position themselves at a desk or even deal with their body appropriately in gymnastics.

Paired reading   A shared reading exercise with child and adult. The adult can drop out when it is felt that the child has a good 'flow' and then come in again if the flow ebbs a little at any time.

Perception   The process of organizing and interpreting the information received through the senses.

Perseveration   Tendency to continue repeating sounds, symbols or activities inappropriately immediately after relevant usage in speech or in writing.

Phoneme   Smallest unit of speech sounds. It may correspond to a single letter (e.g. b, g) or digraph (sh, th, ai, oy).

Phonetics   The study of speech sound, its manner and method of production and representation by written symbols, as in the International Phonetic Alphabet.

Phonics   An approach to reading instruction where the emphasis is placed upon the sound value of letters as a means of word recognition.

Pictogram   A picture which represents a letter or letter sequence.

Proprioception   Feedback to the brain about sensations in the body and unrelated movement from muscles to joint receptors.

Psychosomatic   Generally pertaining to that which is presumed to have both mental and bodily components. The individual may be considerably physically disabled, in the case of gastric ulcers for example, and yet stress and anxiety may play a major part in the generation of the condition and its eventual management.

Reading age   An individual's attainment in reading expressed against the reading standard for the average child in a particular age group.

Reversal   The turning back to front of a letter or word, e.g. 'd' for 'b', 'was' for 'saw'.

Scanning   Glancing quickly through a text to find specific items of information.

Semantic   Referring to the meaning of a morpheme, word, phrase or sentence.

Sensory   Pertaining very generally to the senses, the sense organs, the sense receptors, the afferent neural pathways, sense data, etc.

Sensory discrimination – differential responding to different stimuli
Sensory integration – the neurological process of integrating incoming data from the various sensory channels, e.g. selecting and picking up an object following an auditory command, requires auditory analysis and interpretation leading to visual–motor activity.

Sight word   A word that is not phonetically regular or recognizable by application of spelling rules, e.g. said, once.

Skimming   A method of reading quickly to gain the overall sense of a text.

Spatial orientation   A person's awareness of how their body relates to the environment.

Spelling age   As for *reading age*.

Standardized   A test is said to be standardized when it has been administered to a representative population and its *consistency* and *validity* have proved satisfactory.

Tactile   The ability to interpret sensory stimuli experienced through the sense of touch.

Tracking   The visual pursuit of a stimulus in a prescribed manner, e.g. searching in a left–right direction along a line to pick out a particular letter.

Validity   The extent to which a test measures the area it sets out to test.

Vestibular system   Receptors within the inner ear which react to movement that provides feedback to the brain on the quality of movement produced.

Visual acuity   The capacity to see the fine details of objects in the visual field. In clinical practice standard displays are used, for example the Snellen Chart, allowing for the measurement of the eye's capacity to discriminate fine detail.

Visual perception   The identification, organization and interpretation of sensory data received through the eyes. It may be divided into separate features as follows:

Discrimination – the ability to discern similarities and differences within visually presented material
Closure – the ability to identify a visual stimulus from an incomplete visual presentation
Figure–ground – the ability to perceive objects in the foreground and background and to separate them meaningfully
Memory – the storage of visually presented information long enough to analyse and recall it accurately
Motor planning – the ability to reproduce from memory physical activities which have been previously demonstrated
Sequencing – reproduction of information in the correct order

Vocabulary   The number of words a child can recognize or use in speech or in written form.

Index

Page numbers in **bold** refer to figures and page numbers appearing in *italic* refer to tables.

Headteachers *cont'd*
  working with parents 236–43, 258, 259
Hearing disorders
  and language acquisition 29, 39–40, 256–7
  paediatric evaluation 149
Hearing tests 78
Hereditary factors in dyslexia 147–8, 155, 169, 237
History, classteaching 218
Holiday projects
  classteaching 217
  parents' role 239–40
Homework
  and divorced parents 179
  parents' role 239–40
  policy on 227–8
  problems with 200
Housing, effects of 172
Hyperactive Children's support Group (HASCG) 156
Hyperactivity
  characterization 103
  and dyspraxia 107
  see also Attention deficit hyperactive disorder
Hypermetropia 131–2, 133–4, 135
Hypoactivity, characterization 103

Ideation 106, 107–8, 109–10, 111
IEPs (individual education plans) 185–6
Illinois Test of Psycholinguistic Ability (ITPA) 45
Inattentiveness, see Attention skills
Individual education plans (IEPs) 185–6
Individual tuition, remedial teaching 185, 187–8, 206
Information gathering, by headteachers 234
Information processing 25–7
  adolescents and young adults 35
  and attention deficit disorder 47–8
  classteaching and remediation 198, 204–5
  disorders in 103–4
  educational profile 198

hidden deficits 27–8
mid-school patterns 33–4
neurological factors 40, 148
preschool patterns 29, 39–40
remedial teaching 187
soft signs of dyslexia 47
verbal–performance discrepancies 42–3, 74
vocabulary and comprehension 44–7
and WISC III 38
and writing 117
see also Speech and language therapy
Information technology
  in classteaching 215–16, 218–21
  in remedial teaching 186, 189–90
  resource allocation 235
Intelligence, multiple intelligences concept 232
Intelligence quotient (IQ)
  and attention deficit disorder 48
  early school patterns 32
  and impact of dyslexia 42
  verbal–performance discrepancies 42–3, 74
  WISC III measure 38

Jordan Left–Right Reversal Test 102

Kinaesthetic sense 105, 267
  motor planning 109
  touch typing 219
  in writing 115, 208, 210

LADDER, address 156
Language development and acquisition 28–9, 32, 39–40, 72–3, 170–1, 256–7
  see also Speech and language therapy
Language Master 87–8
Language-related information processing 26–8
  and classteaching 198, 204–5
  multidisciplinary case study 258–9
  neurological factors 40, 148
  preschool patterns 29, 39–40
  remedial teaching 187